PRAISE FOR *A DIM PROGNOSIS*

'This is a brave, funny and heart-rendingly sad diagnosis of our health system, delivered from the trenches. Every healthcare worker in Aotearoa will feel seen by this extraordinary debut memoir. It is startling in its bravery at a time when our healthcare workers are struggling to deliver safe and effective patient care while being gaslit by non-clinical decision makers, who suggest we could simply work harder, with fewer resources, to meet arbitrary targets that look good on paper and do nothing to address decades of underinvestment in health.

'A copy should be delivered to every politician elected to serve the people of this country; it does more than any spreadsheet could possibly do to explain the desperate state of our healthcare system.'

DR EMMA WEHIPEIHANA, *THERE'S A CURE FOR THIS*

'This no-holds-barred account of the New Zealand health service, delivered through the experiences of a doctor in training, is a must-read for all who care about the future of publicly funded healthcare in Aotearoa. At times scathing, the author's observations and critiques reveal a system stifled and constrained by its own rigidity in the face of underfunding, micro-management and overwhelming workloads.'

DR DAVID GALLER, *THINGS THAT MATTER*

A Dim Prognosis

OUR HEALTH SYSTEM IN CRISIS — AND A DOCTOR'S VIEW ON HOW TO FIX IT

IVOR POPOVICH

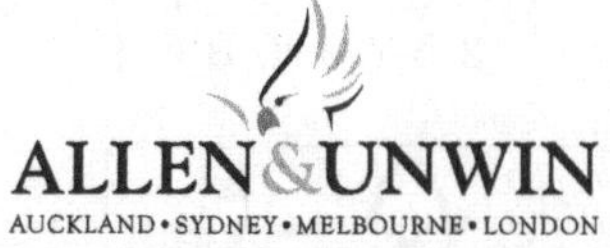

Author's note: To protect the privacy of individuals, some names and identifying details have been changed, and stories have been amalgamated. Events are told to the best of my recollection. Some of the medical conditions and situations described are common, and resemblances to readers' experiences are likely coincidental.

First published in 2025

Allen & Unwin Aotearoa New Zealand
Level 2, 10 College Hill, Freemans Bay
Auckland 1011, New Zealand
+64 (9) 377 3800
auckland@allenandunwin.com
www.allenandunwin.co.nz

83 Alexander Street
Crows Nest NSW 2065, Australia
+61 (2) 8425 0100

EU Authorised Representative: Easy Access System Europe, Mustamäe tee 50, 10621 Tallinn, Estonia, gpsr.requests@easproject.com

A catalogue record for this book is available from the National Library of New Zealand.

ISBN 978 1 991142 41 2

Design by Megan van Staden
Set in FreightText Pro
Cover photograph by Stephen Tilley
Printed and bound in Australia by the Opus Group

3 5 7 9 10 8 6 4

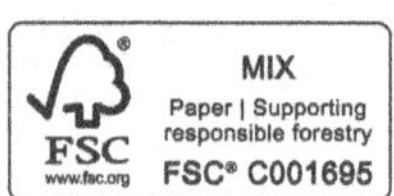

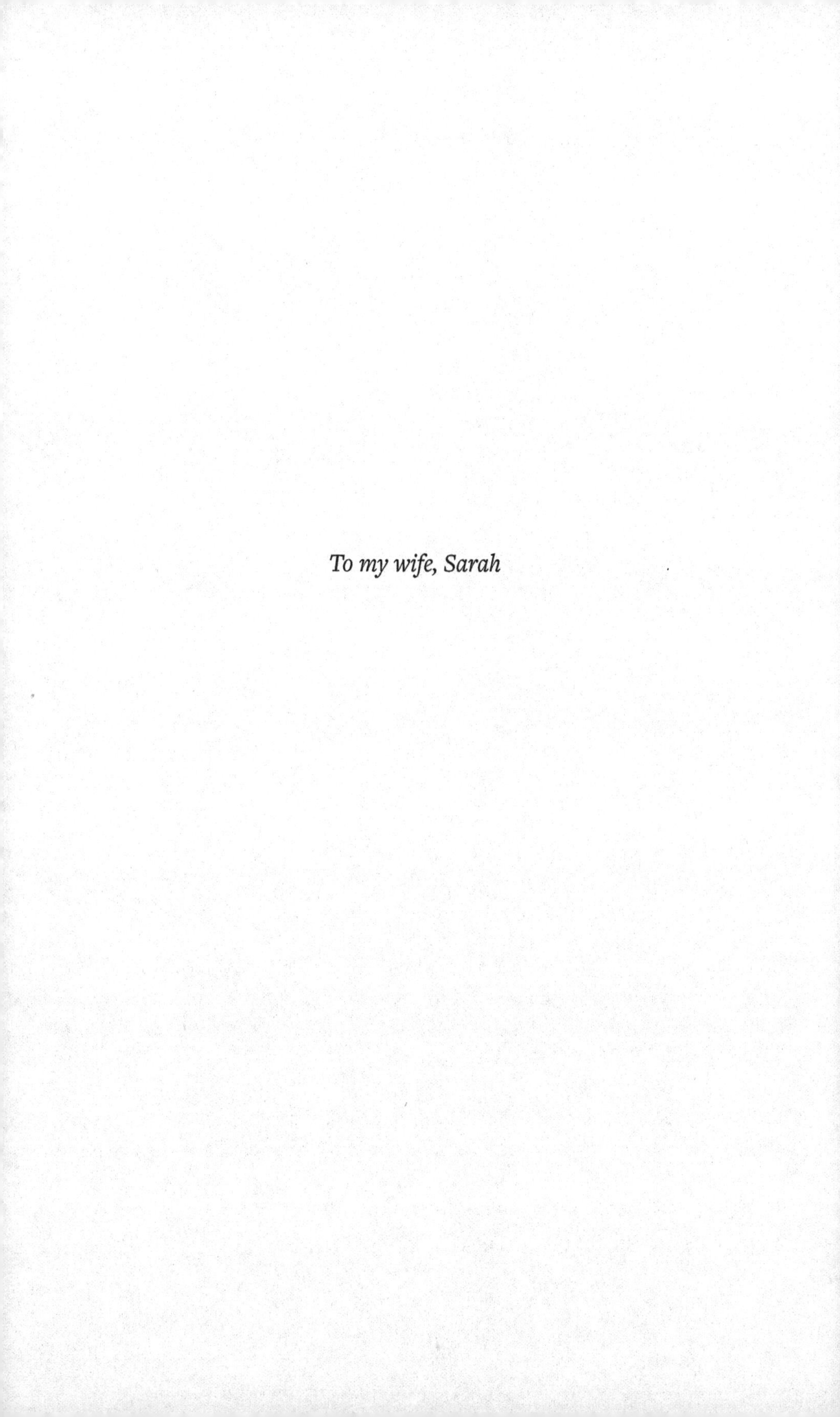

To my wife, Sarah

CONTENTS

1.

ULTRASOUND, NEEDLE, WIRE, DILATOR, LINE, SUTURES

Monday 9 December 2019 started off quite pleasantly. I am not a morning person but I didn't feel my usual lethargy on getting out of bed. I even made time for breakfast, and I bared my teeth at the mirror after brushing them, rating their whiteness. I smoothed out the crinkles on the shoulders of my shirt.

Today was doctor changeover day, when all the registrars change rotations and go to different hospitals. As a registrar in intensive care I was excited because for the first time ever, I wasn't rostered to start straight away on nights. The day shifts early on in a rotation generally went to registrars from other specialties doing stints in the ICU for experience. They needed to attend several days of orientation first, while the familiar hands like me got straight to work — at night.

This time there happened to be more than the usual number of experienced ICU trainees, and I had got lucky. I looked forward to three days of getting paid to hang around, listen to some introductory talks, saunter around the hospital and meet new colleagues. There was certain to be some free food involved as well. I had prepared a list of 'interesting' facts about me in case of an ice-breaker exercise. They made me feel like the most boring person in the world.

The summer smells of hot pavement, cut grass and salty breeze had set in only a few days earlier. I contemplated wearing shorts but decided this might not make the right first impression.

The hospital I was rotating to had the country's

main burns ICU. I had some trepidation, as these were the only types of patient I had not so far seen during my training. I had read up about burns to prepare. The only information I seemed to retain was to cover people in cling-film to reduce heat loss and evaporation. You would think a burn victim had had enough heat, but actually hypothermia after a burn is a major problem because the skin is the main regulator of body temperature.

I tried to memorise how different types of burn looked. First-degree was basically sunburn. Second-degree was paler, blistery and moist. Third-degree burns were white and leathery.

After I arrived I sat chatting with the other registrars in the ICU meeting room. My friend Drew was starting with me. It's always nice to have someone familiar around, and I kept looking at the door waiting for him to arrive. The door burst open at exactly 8.30, but it wasn't Drew. It was the director of the unit.

'Lovely to meet you all,' he said. 'We'll get to know each other in a second, but first of all I have some bad news. Drew is rostered to be on night shift tonight . . .'

Ah, that's right, I said to myself. I'd forgotten he wouldn't be at orientation.

'. . . but unfortunately he's stuck in Timaru and can't get out because of landslides caused by the flooding down there. He's okay!' he swiftly clarified, 'but the roads are blocked. So that means whoever's rostered for night relief is going to have to fill in.'

I leaned my chair back on its legs, put my hands behind

my head and smiled smugly. Thank god that wasn't me.

The director peered at a clipboard in his hand.

'Ivor. Looks like you're rostered as night relief. Sorry, bud.'

The front of my chair fell to Earth with a dull sound. I gaped at the director.

'Oh. Right . . . I didn't . . . I didn't realise. So do I stay here now?'

'Well, why don't you stay for quick introductions, then come down with everyone to the security office to get your ID. Then you should go home and get some sleep, and we'll see you at 8 p.m.!'

Just fucking great. I wanted to shake my fist at the sky, at this great cosmic joke being played on me. The Lord giveth, then taketh away.

◆◆◆

I lay awake at midday, staring at the ceiling in my room with the blinds down. Usually I could sleep in the middle of an earthquake if I needed to, but the build-up and let-down of the day kept my eyes wide open. I tried counting sheep, then cows, then I put on some meditative music. Finally I managed to drift off into some hazy, restless hallucination where I was running away from the police through the hospital corridors because I had accidentally prescribed someone a kilogram of morphine.

The sound of chirping birds from my phone woke me. I stabbed at the Dismiss icon with my index finger, missing a few times before I finally got it. I pondered that technology was not only taking over nature, but making us despise its sounds.

I flicked on the telly as I stirred my cup of tea. And dropped my spoon to the ground.

A faint, jagged outline broke the perfectly straight horizon line. From it billowed a colossal white and black plume, filling most of the camera shot. It ballooned and deformed like a demon reaching down and trying to envelop the sea. Despite everything roiling above it, the water remained tranquil and blue.

Whakaari White Island, an active offshore volcano in the Bay of Plenty, had erupted while being visited by dozens of tourists. I remember loudly saying 'Holy shit!', and wishing I had managed to get in more sleep. It might be a long night.

I was glued to the news for the next hour, watching the disaster unfold. The newscasters solemnly reported new developments about every 10 minutes. First, it was unknown how many people had been on the island when it erupted. Then came reports of over a hundred people injured. That was soon updated to 30–40.

Injured victims, most badly burned, were transported by passing tour boats to the wharf in Whakatāne. There, they were triaged and treated on scene by paramedics before being sent to Whakatāne Hospital. This many critical patients all at once would have been a huge deal for even the biggest hospitals in the country, let alone a small rural hospital. They must have been overwhelmed.

Generally in summer I drive to work with the windows down and music blaring. This day I drove in silence.

In the ICU the atmosphere hung thick like the clouds over the ocean in the images that were being shown on every screen.

The specialist on call that day, and until eight the next morning, was Elijah, a short man with a booming voice who was wearing shorts and a Hawaiian shirt, quite at odds with the seriousness of the day's events.

'So, Ivor, have you done any ICU before?'

'Some,' I said.

'Good, good. Well, buckle up, my friend.'

Patients were being offloaded from Whakatāne Hospital to burn units and trauma centres around the country. That was us.

I was one of two registrars on that night. I was assigned to look after the patients in the unit, while my colleague Liz would field referrals from wards, theatres and the emergency department. Usually the specialist would conduct an evening ward round just after 8 p.m., make plans for the night, then disappear to bed but remain available to be called if we needed them.

'The first priority,' Elijah told us, 'is to free up some space, and get some of our patients to other hospitals. Liz, we'll need to try to keep any new surgical patients in theatres, or in the recovery room overnight, and any patients in ED or the ward that are not too unstable might need to be transferred to other units if possible.'

The first hour of the night was spent organising

ambulance transfers to other ICUs in the city. All the while we waited; troops lining the trenches, disquieted by the silence, knowing it was the kind of silence you heard when the enemy's artillery guns stopped firing — not a comfort but just a sign that the main wave of the attack was about to come over the hill.

More pictures came through, from the island itself. Rocky hills and flat ground all covered with a thick white-grey ash that from a distance almost looked like snow. A tour helicopter had been blasted off its landing pad and sat with its rotor blades bent crooked like the legs of a spider.

The pager beeped, and Elijah and Liz went down to the ED to receive the first Whakaari patient. I waited. The lights in the main ICU corridor had been switched off.

It was a while before they arrived back in the unit. The patient was unconscious with a breathing tube in. I scanned their body for the tell-tale signs of third-degree burns but there was not much to see. They were covered head to toe in padded white dressings. The face and lips were wet and swollen and blistered. You lose masses of body water through badly burnt skin, and this leads to severe dehydration, causing low blood pressure and depriving the vital organs of blood supply. Elijah and Liz had resuscitated the patient with intravenous fluid but their blood pressure was still dangerously low.

'We need a central line,' Elijah said to me.

Patients with severe burns often need litres and litres of intravenous fluid in the first 24 hours to keep them hydrated — sometimes more than 20 litres. We also needed to infuse a powerful medication that would tighten up the blood vessels and combat the shock caused by the burn. This medication needed to go through a long line placed in one of the body's big veins, either the jugular vein in the neck or the femoral vein in the groin. This patient would also need multiple other infusions over time — too many to deliver through smaller lines in the arms or hands, which were in any case too burnt to find good veins.

I wheeled the procedure trolley in. There was not much clear skin in the neck, but there was unexpectedly healthy skin over the waist and upper thighs, like an underwear tan line. We would later come to realise that even light clothing had offered protection against the heat, and victims' underwear had shielded that part of the body. It would become a common site from which to take skin grafts for these patients.

I laid out all my equipment on the trolley, painted the groin with pink-violet sterilising solution, and started to scrub up into a surgical gown, hat, mask and gloves. I used ultrasound on the thigh to locate the femoral vein, then it was in with the needle. A flash of blood back into the syringe, then carefully threading a slender stainless-steel wire through the needle. Needle out, wire still in place, then over the wire and through the skin with a thick plastic dilator. The skin crackled slightly as it separated. Dilator out, the line itself then sliding over the wire up to the hilt, then wire out, and stitching the line into place.

Beads of sweat started to accumulate on my forehead and roll down the bridge of my nose. I desperately wanted to scratch it. The sterile gowns did not breathe very well, and the room was warmed up to 32°C to stop the patient becoming hypothermic. An acrid, sulphurous smell had started to roll up under my nostrils.

When I was done, no sooner had I scooped the surgical hat off my head and thrown it into the bin, my hair sticking up into the air from all the sweat, than Elijah rolled in with another patient.

'Needs a central line. The surgeon is coming up to do escharotomies [surgical treatment of full-thickness burns that go all the way around a limb].'

I opened a new sterile pack and put on another lot of stuffy gear.

Same deal: ultrasound, needle, wire, dilator, line, sutures. Now I was smelling my own breath behind the mask, mixed in with everything.

The nurses called me back to the first patient, whose blood pressure was dropping. We squeezed more intravenous fluid into their veins and the BP began to recover. Someone tugged on the back of my scrubs. It was Elijah.

'Liz is off seeing a patient on the ward. Come down to ED with me.'

We jogged along the corridor and down a back staircase to the ED resus bay. Another Whakaari patient had arrived, this time not intubated. They had deteriorated dramatically during the flight over and were practically unconscious, with a blood pressure that could barely be recorded.

'I'll intubate; you get ready to do another line.'

By this point sweat was starting to soak through the front of my scrubs.

The burns surgical team arrived. Quick introductions.

'First day?' they asked me.

'That's right,' I said.

'Welcome.'

'Thanks.'

Ultrasound, needle, wire, dilator, line, sutures.

With more intravenous fluid and drugs we slowly pulled the patient's blood pressure back up to a safe level. This patient had dressings applied very loosely and the surgical team peeled them off to look underneath. What I saw was unlike anything I had seen in the textbooks. The patient was embedded — front, back, arms and legs — in volcanic ash, black as coal. I couldn't tell the depth of the burn wounds underneath. Spots of cherry-red burn peeked out from under the ash here and there.

The surgical team's blue nitrile gloves started disintegrating on contact with the ash. They kept having to don new gloves. What kind of nasty shit is in that ash? I wondered. My throat had started to feel a bit scratchy.

'I'll stay down here,' said Elijah. 'Why don't you head back up to the ICU, they're just going up to do the escharotomies now.'

One of the surgeons was getting set up. When a third-degree burn goes all the way around a limb, the thick burn scar can cut off the blood supply. The surgeon unravelled the dressing on the patient's arms and started cutting with his scalpel from the shoulder all the way down to the fingertips, to release the scar. The fingertips, which had been cold and pale, started warming up.

Some details were starting to emerge. There had been three groups of victims on the island: a group standing right near the crater, a group halfway back to the boats near a rocky outcropping, and a group near the helicopter that had been blown off its landing pad, close to the water but exposed. We didn't know it at this stage, but everyone in the first group perished. Those in the third group had worse burns than the second group, who were closer to the eruption but able to shelter behind rocks.

When we heard that the victims had been doused with seawater for first aid before they were transported to Whakatāne Hospital, Elijah and I looked at each other sideways. This was life-saving, but we wondered what kind of bacteria might have been lurking in the seawater and whether we had to worry about infection this early on.

'We need to figure out who's had what scans,' Elijah told me. 'Remember, a burn patient is first and foremost a trauma patient.'

Whakaari exploded when underground water was heated by passing magma and flashed to steam, bursting outwards in a superheated cloud of acidic ash that travelled at lightning speed. Fragments of rock, flung around like whizzing bullets, could damage internal organs the same way as in a car crash. Some of the patients had had CT scans at other hospitals to look for such injuries; others hadn't.

I sat at a tiny desk flicking through pages of photocopied documents written in chicken-scratch, trying to figure out who had had what. A unified electronic system would have made this child's play, but we didn't have that (and still don't). I searched for blood results. I searched for records of how much fluid they had been given before arriving to us, what procedures had been carried out, what drugs had been given.

It was all a goddamn mess. A job that would have taken 15 minutes with good technology instead took several valuable hours. All the while new patients kept arriving, and I ran around sticking in central lines all night long.

Ultrasound, needle, wire, dilator, line, sutures.

Ultrasound, needle, wire, dilator, line, sutures.

Ultrasound, needle, wire, dilator, line, sutures.

We kept being called back to the early patients, who were becoming increasingly unstable. More fluid, more drugs. Surgeons were running around all over the place, whipping patients off to the operating room to scrub down volcanic ash and release scars that were suffocating limbs.

An added difficulty was that we didn't know who most of the patients were. They were unidentified other than by their room number. It was an ICU full of ash-covered, mummified identical siblings.

At one point I stood frozen in the middle of the ICU, not knowing where to go to next. It felt as if we were trying to hold on to an expanding mist with our hands. I was sweat-soaked from head to toe and feeling the nausea you get when you haven't eaten for hours.

Mostly, I felt as if we were alone. We were on a tiny fishing vessel in the North Sea, in the middle of the night, miles from shore, with freak waves breaking against our hull and the wind howling something terrible. At any moment a wave could tip us over and we would be lost forever at sea, no one to hear our mayday call, no one coming to rescue us.

I thought about something Elijah had said to me at some point in the night. 'These patients have been a lot more unstable than your average burn victim. And what's interesting is that they've all had their burn percentage upgraded since arriving to us. I mean, estimating burn percentage is a tricky business, and non-burn centres will always be off by a little, but they've been consistently under on everybody. And by quite a bit. There's something unusual about whatever is in this ash.'

It was an observation we had no time to ponder.

One of the nurses approached and handed me a printout.

'Doctor, this patient's calcium seems to be falling.'

I looked down at the sheet of paper, blinking. My eyes were blurring.

'Yeah, that is pretty low. Let's give some calcium chloride.'

'Bed 3's was also low. Dr Elijah just prescribed some calcium for him too.'

'Is that right?'

Those two patients were the least stable.

I walked into Room 3 where Elijah was seated at the computer sucking on an ice-block he had raided from the paediatric fridge.

'Did you see that Bed 4 has a low calcium as well?'

He stopped mid-lick and looked up at me with narrowed eyes.

'There's some weird metabolic effect going on here. Start them both on calcium infusions.'

One of the patients arrived back from the operating room, accompanied by their anaesthetist. We went to take a handover.

'He got really unstable halfway through. He had a low calcium on the gas [a blood gas is a type of blood test] and replacing it seemed to be associated with a big improvement, more than I would normally expect.'

'Yeah, we've just put two patients on calcium infusions.'

The anaesthetist stroked his goateed chin.

'You don't think . . . we don't think we're dealing with hydrofluoric acid, do we?'

'Hydrofluoric acid?'

'Yeah, it's behaving like hydrofluoric acid poisoning. I think you find it in volcanoes.'

We all whipped out our phones to start googling and soon confirmed that hydrofluoric acid is indeed found in volcanic ash.

Hydrofluoric acid burns are usually associated with industrial accidents. The fluorine component combines with calcium in the body to form calcium fluoride, which takes away calcium that the heart needs to pump effectively. As volcanic burns are extremely rare, there was no one in the world at that stage who could call themselves an expert in them.

Soon most of our Whakaari patients were on calcium infusions. But we soon realised something even more important. The burnt tissue was acting as a reservoir of corrosive acids, including hydrofluoric acid, leaching calcium out of the tissues underneath and dissolving them. Until the burnt tissue was cut out, the burn would keep getting deeper and it would keep releasing fluoride ions into the bloodstream.

Usually you have 24–48 hours to cut out a burn, in an operation called debridement. Debridement can result in a lot of blood loss. Do it too early, while the patient is still being resuscitated and while they are unstable, and they may not survive. Now the surgeons needed to get in and debride an ICU full of patients as soon as they could.

Multiple operating theatres ran 24/7 for that whole first week. Thereafter, the surgeons would continually take patients back to theatre to discover that tissue they had left clean and healthy and ready for grafting was now leaden and boggy, and needed further debridement.

I was called back to the patient in Bed 7, who had been deteriorating all night. They had a 90 per cent burn. We had thrown everything we had at them. Thirty litres of fluid, multiple powerful medications to keep the blood pressure up, a steroid medication, a paralytic drug and careful adjustments of the ventilator to try to get enough oxygen into the lungs, which were charred by the ash they had sucked in.

An archaic rule of thumb is that a patient's likelihood of mortality is their age plus the percentage burn. Going by that rule, our patient had no chance. In the era of modern burn care this is no longer used, but it was a sober reminder of what we were up against.

The patient's blood pressure was 50/20.

Elijah breathed out a large sigh and flung his pen at the wall. It ricocheted off the wall and into the rubbish bin.

'Have we located any family?' he asked the nurse.

'No.'

'It's time to stop. This is unsurvivable.'

◆◆◆

Eventually 8 a.m. rolled around. Somehow our little boat had made it to land, but it was to dock there only briefly. Tonight we would set off into the tempest again.

I drove home, and fell asleep as soon as I hit the sheets.

At 8 p.m. I was back. I overheard the nurses talking about a kid who had died on the first night. I interrupted their conversation.

'Um, I think you're mistaken. Only one person died last night and it was an adult.'

'Oh. You haven't heard? The police identified the patient today. It was a child.'

I went into the toilet and wept.

2.

WELCOME TO THE JUNGLE

A handy guide to the hospital hierarchy

House officer/intern: a doctor in their first year or two after graduation who rotates around to a different specialty every three months.

Junior doctor: a blanket term for any doctor who is not a qualified specialist.

Locum: a doctor of any level who is hired temporarily to fill a gap in the roster.

Registrar: a junior doctor at least three years out from graduation, working in a particular specialty.

RMO (registered medical officer): another term for a junior doctor.

SMO (senior medical officer): another term for a specialist.

Specialist/consultant: a doctor who has completed training with one of the Australasian specialist medical colleges.

Surgeon: a consultant who specialised in surgery.

My first-ever day as a doctor, starting on orthopaedics, I clipped a pager on to my belt and felt important. Within a few hours of its incessant beeping I realised that being important means being needed, and that sometimes it would be nice not to be needed.

One of the pages asked me to review the results of a patient's urine test. I sat down at the computer and read the following:

MSU
WBC: 60
RBC: 10
Epi: <10

I looked sideways at the other house officer, also on her first day.

'I know that in order to diagnose a UTI [urinary tract infection] you need white cells [WBC] in the urine. And an absence of epithelial cells, to make sure the sample is not contaminated. But how many white cells is too many?'

She stared blankly back. Then at my computer screen.

'Umm, dunno. Sixty seems like a lot, right?'

'Yeah, but I remember seeing a result once that had over a thousand. So . . .'

Silence.

'Let's ask our registrar.'

We got the following helpful reply: 'I'm about to scrub into theatre, do you think I have time to answer amateur fucking questions like that? Why don't you guys figure it out?'

The patient received antibiotics they didn't actually need.

◆◆◆

Later that week our team was looking after a patient whose bones were infected with *Staphylococcus aureus*, a common bacterium that lives on the skin. The bug had seeped into his bloodstream and was making him very unwell. In fact, unbeknown to us, his major organs were starting to shut down. My pager buzzed and it was the nurses telling me his blood pressure was starting to get dangerously low. I turned to the orthopaedic consultant.

'I've just been told Mr X's BP is down to 85/50.'

He raised his brows, then started flicking both outstretched hands rapidly towards me.

'So go! Sort it out!'

I arrived breathless to find Mr X looking sweaty and pale.

I recalled that the treatment of low blood pressure when a person has sepsis is IV fluid to fill up the heart and allow it to eject more blood with each beat. Then I saw that his IV line had fallen out. I struggled for half an hour to insert another. His veins kept rolling and slipping off to the side — it was like trying to stab a single noodle with a fork. I just knew the nurses were rolling their eyes at me as I asked to be passed another IV, then another, then another.

Once it was in, we got a litre into him and his blood pressure came up. But our success was short-lived. Sepsis is an unpredictable condition, and treating low blood pressure with fluid can be an ethereal enterprise. Like a breath of air on a winter morning, whose mist hangs suspended for just a bit, then dissipates.

So he received another litre. Then another. There's that famous line: 'Insanity is doing the same thing over and over again and expecting different results.'

I called the orthopaedic consultant.

'I'm in clinic.'

'I know but I need help.' I filled him in briefly. 'What else can I do for this man?'

'Well, he's on flucloxacillin [an antibiotic], isn't he?'

'Yes.'

'Well, that's all good then. Just carry on with that.'

I was down having lunch a few hours later and my phone rang. Back in the days of pagers, this was unusual.

'Hello?'

'Hello, this is the infectious diseases registrar. I'm reviewing Mr X because of his positive blood cultures.'

A moment of silence, then he continued. 'I'm standing in front of a very sick man.'

The sudden realisation that you've fucked up is the same feeling as turning around in a crowded mall and realising you can't find your child. One week in and I've already been tossed out of the ring, I thought.

'You need to call ICU. In fact, you know what . . . I'll call them. You just . . . just let your boss know.'

◆◆◆

I was sitting in the orthopaedic handover room one morning. The registrar was handing over all the patients they had admitted overnight, who would be seen that morning by the consultant (specialist) on call and their team. Each team consists of a consultant, a registrar, and usually a couple of house officers/interns. House officers are in their first year or two post graduation and rotate around to a different specialty every three months. Their job is to do the boring and time-consuming tasks nobody else wants to do. This was me.

The overnight registrar was describing a patient with a hand injury. The consultant turned down the corners of his lips.

'Did you do an X-ray?'

'N-no.'

'Why the fuck not? Do I look like I have X-ray vision? Do I look like fucking Superman to you?'

'No, sir. I just . . . well, it was just an infected wound. I didn't think . . .' He trailed off to an embarrassed silence in front of a room of 30 people, with all the orthopaedic teams in attendance.

'Furthermore . . . you've written on this handover sheet that the wound came about when she pricked herself on a *wild hedgehog*.'

'Yes, that's right.'

'What the fuck is a wild hedgehog? All hedgehogs are wild, you imbecile. Have you ever seen a domesticated hedgehog wandering around on a leash? Well? Have you? With a little collar saying "My name is Spot, return me to this address if lost"?'

'I'm sorry. It was a hedgehog, just a hedgehog.'

'Right, well, that's the handover finally done. Now, which registrar is operating with me today?'

A man sitting next to me piped up. 'I am.'

The consultant looked at him for a split second with a snarl of his lips, then turned his entire body away from him.

'I ask again, who is operating with me today?'

At least his abuse was only verbal, unlike one of his colleagues. You could tell his pal had been forced to attend an anger management course by the painful contortion of his facial muscles when he was interacting with someone he figured he should probably try to be nice to.

◆◆◆

This would not be a very interesting book if I focused on the swathes of nice and normal people who make their living as hospital doctors. But the first step in addressing issues in the health system is to put your own house in order. We have a culture problem. Culture problems exist partly because big egos gravitate to medicine, but mostly because the work environment sculpts people into grotesque carvings.

The world of inpatient medicine can be divided into surgery and general medicine. Surgeons like to believe they are the only ones treating fixable problems; what can be cut away with a knife is fixable. Prescribing someone who has been ravaged by a monster stroke an aspirin a day doesn't quite have the same appeal. Medics, on the other hand, regard themselves as 'thinkers' and see surgeons as blunt tools who don't know how to manage simple medical problems like diabetes.

We could speculate that the origins of the divide hark back to the old days when surgery was performed by barbers. In fact the Hippocratic Oath specifically forbids physicians from taking up the knife and performing surgery. This is the reason surgeons revert to being called Mr or Ms rather than Dr once they qualify as specialists.

On top of that, the various medical specialties themselves are akin to high-school cliques. These divisions go back a long way, but the tribalism among hospital doctors is certainly fuelled by the conditions they work under.

Doctors can spend up to 70 hours a week at work, sometimes even longer. Your shifts can be 14 hours long and the pressure incessant. In the face of the erosion of your sleep habits, hobbies and personal relationships, you have two options. You can become a miserable misanthrope, or you can convince yourself that you belong to a special group of people who are more important and skilled than anyone else. Or both.

There is also the unavoidable human response that you grow to resent whoever makes work for you. And they make a lot of work for each other. Medics, when their patients have co-existent problems that might require a surgical consultation, and vice versa. This is why everybody craps on ED doctors. About 90 per cent of the patients who come to hospital are dealt with by the emergency department. However, this is invisible to other doctors in the hospital, who see only the 10 per cent that are referred on; so as far as they are concerned, the only function of an ED doctor is to create work for them.

At one point in my life I was the medical registrar on call. ('On call' means different things in different contexts. A consultant may be at home on call 'after hours', whereas a registrar on call is more likely working a shift and/or being the contact person for referrals and advice at the same time.)

My phone rang.

'Hello, this is the med reg,' I answered.

'Oh, hey man, it's Ben from the ED. Got a referral for you.'

No matter how appropriate the referral, this sentence is always met with a spasm of annoyance, even if it's your best friend on the other end of the line and taking referrals is your job.

'Go on.'

'Well, I've got this 70-year-old woman who blacked out while driving her car. She crashed and has sustained fractures to her anterior ribs 7 through 11 on the right, and, ah, some ribs on the left as well. She also has some transverse spinous process fractures of the lumbar spine. I discussed with ortho — no precautions needed for that.

Rest of the pan scan, including C spine, is normal. Anyway, ECG shows—'

'That sounds like pretty major trauma. Shouldn't she be under the surgeons?'

'Well, yeah, probably. I talked to them, but they said she needs work-up for the cause of her blackout, so should go under you guys. They're happy to consult.'

I bet they are, I thought to myself. It's much easier to make someone else do the time-consuming work of writing up the admission notes, prescribing all the medications, following up all the blood tests and generally assuming responsibility for the patient. Any chance to punt a patient to another service and reduce your own workload is a game-winning kick. And in such a game, the general medical service represents the kiddie goalpost.

Sometimes you need to put up a fight in the best interests of the patient.

'Nah, mate, I'm not admitting a trauma patient under medicine. Get the surgical registrar to call me.'

A few minutes later the phone rang again.

'Hey, it's gen surg here. You wanted to talk about Ms X?'

'Yeah, you guys need to admit this woman. She's broken like half her ribs. She's a trauma patient.'

'But we need to know why she blacked out, and you guys need to work her up for that.'

'The work-up is pretty simple. She needs an ECG and some monitoring. And an X-ray, which she's already had. And you have scanned her head already too. I'm happy to consult, but the medical wards don't know how to take care of trauma patients.'

'Well, we're not very good at working up collapses.'

'All she needs is telemetry [monitoring of heart rhythm by a portable device], which can be done on any ward. Hell, I'll do the telemetry request for you. But rib fractures, anaesthetic blocks, potentially an epidural — medicine can't manage those.'

'If there's a cardiac cause for her collapse, that's the more serious issue.'

'But poor pain management is the thing that might kill her at this stage. I'm not admitting this patient to medicine.'

◆◆◆

It sounds antithetical to the ideals of medicine to be playing hot potato with patients. Sometimes it's because you truly believe a patient is best served by being under the care of another specialty. Sometimes it's because you are so stretched you truly don't know where you will find the time to see another patient. Occasionally it's because someone is being a lazy bastard.

Well, as lazy as you can be while working a 70-hour week.

Unless you're a hermit you will have seen in the news that New Zealand hospitals are overcrowded and at breaking point. In fact they have been this way for as long as I can remember. When I had appendicitis as a teenager

I was laid on a stretcher in a corridor while I waited to be seen. Lifting my head to look around made my belly tense up, sending a surge of agony through my body, so I had to lie flat. My eyes rolled back and forth, tracking the bustling traffic in the corridor. A lady in a nice pant suit. Who was she? Someone important. She carried a tail of earnest-looking people in scrubs carrying clipboards, trying to keep up.

A tired-looking Middle Eastern doctor was talking to a patient further down. Their voices carried right along the corridor.

'You know if you keep smoking, you're going to keep having asthma attacks, right?'

'Well, I don't fucking care.'

'All right, well, it's your life, my friend. See you back here next week.'

'Whatever.'

The doctor moved to the next patient, an old man.

'So, my friend, what brings you to hospital?'

'I can't poop.'

'You can't poop, huh? How long have you not pooped for?'

'One month.'

'A month?! You haven't passed a bowel motion for a whole month?'

'That's right.'

'Not even once?'

'No.'

'Where does it all go, man?'

He started cackling and it took him a few seconds to compose himself. I also started laughing, in those little spasms of exhalation that you do when you're trying to stop yourself but just can't. Every laugh caused pain in my abdomen.

The corridor was like a scene from a war movie. Further down, another doctor was breaking the news to a patient that they had found cancer on his scan. Nearby, a janitor was attacking the floor with a large mop. A stressed-looking doctor rushed past him, talking on the phone. As he was walking, his pager started making an enormous racket. He reached for it, in the process knocking a tall skinny container off the janitor's trolley and spilling liquid all over the floor. The intercom was calling loudly for Nurse Smith to report to Room 105 please. A worried woman was stroking the hand of her mother, who lay bundled up in bed sheets on a stretcher next to me. She grabbed the arm of a passing medic. 'We've been waiting four hours; when are we going to see someone?'

3.

YOU GET WHAT YOU PAY FOR

As I've mentioned, most patients' first point of contact with a hospital is the emergency department, where the majority are treated and sent home. So this is many people's only experience of hospital. Given that all public services are beholden to public satisfaction, the ED is the lips of the pig, and enormous attention is applied from time to time to make them nice and juicy and red.

In 2009 the New Zealand government decided it was going to tackle overcrowding in EDs. The six-hour rule for all hospitals introduced a new target to have 95 per cent of ED patients discharged, admitted or transferred within six hours.

Within a few years, the corridor patients had disappeared and ED waiting times had fallen dramatically. A win for government-mandated targets?

At the risk of stating the obvious, the long waits had not been a result of doctors and nurses sitting around on their arses. If you told someone who had just seen 25 patients in a single shift, scarfed down a sandwich on the run and not had a piss since they started work that they could do better if they worked harder and faster, they might well have slapped you right in the face.

What happened was that hospitals diverted resources to making sure the targets would be achieved. New IT systems were introduced to track patients' length of stay in the department. New 'short stay' areas were created in the ED that were exempt from the six-hour rule, to which patients were funnelled if they were about to 'breach'.

Further new areas were created in the hospital — called 'assessment' or 'diagnostic' units — for patients who were clearly going to end up being admitted. They could be punted there after a quick assessment in the ED, to wait to be seen by a doctor. Extra staff were hired.

The problem was temporarily fixed because district health boards did the only thing that worked: invested more money into staffing and beds. They wanted to avoid losing the game — better care was simply a side-effect. Whipping a collapsed horse does not make it run.

As a registrar rotating through general medicine in 2023, I brought up the on-call roster for the day.

'Right, so I'm first call this evening. Second call . . . vacant. Great. Third call also vacant. Perfect.'

'Just you and me, brother,' my colleague Sam said with feigned enthusiasm.

I looked over at him with eyebrows raised.

'I thought they were still paying escalated locum rates for these shifts. Why is nobody picking them up?'

'Because all the locums have picked up night shifts.'

I glanced back at the screen and sure enough, all the (better-paid) night-shift positions were filled. Something caught my eye. 'It says here that Dr Castleman has picked up a night shift! Jesus, the admins can't even tell consultants from registrars. He'll be doing the night shift from his nice warm bed!'

Sam looked at me, unsure whether he should be amused or disappointed at my naiveté.

'Um, dude, they've been doing that for a few months now — putting the on-call consultant's name in one of the boxes so it looks like there's one less vacancy than there is.'

I put my head in my hands.

'Oh well, hell, there's only 20 patients waiting to be seen,' I said sarcastically.

I scanned down the list to work out who had been waiting the longest. Six hours 23 minutes. Five hours 49. Five hours 48. All with chest pain. I hoped none of them were actually having a heart attack.

I zeroed in on an elderly man with chest pain. 'All right, what do we have here?' I said to myself. 'Eighty years old, history of ischaemic heart disease and—'

My phone rang.

'Hey, its ED here. I've got this 30-year-old, no risk factors, chest pain for two hours this morning, ECG all normal, but troponin [a protein found in the cells of the heart] has gone from less than 5 to 6, so the chest pain protocol says they need admitting.' (The lowest lab measure is <5.)

'But that's a normal troponin level.'

'Yeah, but the protocol says a 50 per cent rise needs admission.'

'How is <5 to 6 a 50 per cent rise?'

'It must have been 4, or lower, so that would be at least a 50 per cent increase.'

'Yes, I mean that's true, but that's not really how you're supposed to use that protocol.'

'I don't make the rules. It's your protocol.'

'It's not *my* protocol. It's a stupid protocol. You want me to admit a 30-year-old without risk factors and a normal ECG and troponin when I've got 20 patients waiting to be seen?'

'*I* don't want you to; the protocol says that's what you need to do.'

'Okay, okay, fine, send them over to us.'

I brought up the admission board to add the patient to our expected list. The page wouldn't load. Then the programme crashed. I had to restart it, which took 2 minutes 23 seconds. (I counted.)

As I was entering the details, the phone rang again.

'Hi, it's one the surgical house officers. I have this patient with a potassium of 2.8, because of vomiting, and also low magnesium. Just wanting advice on the best way to replace both of these?'

'Have you talked to the surgical registrar?'

'Umm, no.'

'Why not?' came out more pointedly than intended.

'Well, they're busy in theatre.'

'And I'm busy down here. They should be your first point of call for surgical patients. I can assure you they know how to replace electrolytes just as well as me,' I uttered with increasing staccato.

I heard whimpering on the line and took a deep breath. Was this really the kind of doctor I wanted to be to juniors?

'I'm sorry, I didn't mean to be rude. Look, the best way for this kind of patient . . .' I proceeded with an explanation.

Back to updating the admission board.

The phone rang again. I need to change that ringtone, I thought, because it's really starting to piss me off.

'Hey there, it's ED here. I've got this 100-year-old . . .'

He ran down the story, which was almost immaterial. Everybody knows a person's age is roughly their percentage chance of needing admission. I'm only being half-facetious. Add another 5 per cent for the fact it was after 5 p.m.

'Yup, yup, just put him on our board.'

All right, maybe I could now go and see my 80-year old patient at last . . .

The pager on my belt erupted in a cacophony of beeps.

HYPERACUTE STROKE ED RESUS.

I closed all the tabs and headed over to the resus bay.

A pudgy man sat on the bed staring blankly at me.

'Hold your arms up in the air,' I instructed him. I stuck my arms up to show him.

He nodded with a goofy grin and said, 'Si.'

'I think he's Spanish,' said a colleague.

No shit, Sherlock.

'So what's the neurology?' I asked.

My colleague looked a little taken aback at my directness.

'He was found slumped over outside the supermarket staring into space.'

'How is that a stroke? Does he have anything focal?'

'I'm not sure. I don't think he can understand us and I can't get him to follow any commands.'

I turned back to the patient and thrust my limbs in the air again. He continued staring at me with the same shit-eating grin.

'So as you can see, it's hard to assess him for any focal neurology.'

I grunted, annoyed at my colleague, which I knew was unreasonable. Being annoyed at the patient would be unprofessional. I was annoyed at the world. I wished I believed in God, so I could be annoyed at him.

'His breath stinks of alcohol. Isn't he likely just drunk? What's in his shopping bag over there?'

'A pack of cigarettes, a *TV Guide* and two bottles of wine.'

I raised my eyebrows at him.

'I didn't say they were *empty*, did I? You really want to take the risk here, *Doctor*?'

'No, no. Just do the CT stroke protocol. And flick him over to medicine.'

Here I have become the same disfigured sculpture of myself that I bemoaned in others earlier. Everyone has a threshold where the incessant calls and the inability to feel like you have the time and resources to do the absolute best you can for every single patient gets to you. I had reached mine.

I extricated myself from the resus bay and went to see my 80-year-old. I arrived at Bed 4B to find a crumpled sheet.

A nurse walked by.

'Oh, you looking for that man? He signed a discharge against medical advice about 10 minutes ago. Said he'd rather die at home than spend another hour waiting in this shithole. His words.'

I kept an eye on the newspaper death notices for the next week or two, but saw nothing that matched.

The mute Spaniard turned out not to have had a stroke.

Like in the *Terminator* movies, Judgement Day cannot be prevented, only postponed. It is inevitable. Read that in a thick Austrian accent. The extra resources dumped into the system in the early 2000s could only last so long, and no significant investment has occurred since. In 2025 we are back to where we were, with a much larger population to service.

Every shift I walk down the old ED corridors, with bits of grey showing under the peeling white paint, and I see gurneys pushed up against the walls. Ambulance crew sit next to them on pieces of equipment, waiting for a bed in the ED to become available for their patient. The patients in those beds are waiting for a bed to become available on a ward. More and more patients are pushed into the waiting room of the ED, even those who really should have a bed.

In the ICU, where I now work, patients wait for days for a ward bed. We cancel major high-risk surgeries because there are not enough spaces in the ICU for them to come to after their operation.

We call this bed-block. It is not an ED problem any more than congestion on the motorway is caused by the car at the back of the queue.

We have known since the early 2000s that the population of over-65s in New Zealand is going to double between 2000 and 2030. We also know — and I don't want to sound ageist but it's true — that the elderly use up most of our healthcare resources. That's okay; these people have paid their dues and it is our responsibility to look after them. But we just don't have the means.

We are now getting to the steep part of that rise, and moving faster than initial estimates. Many things in healthcare are complicated, but the following is simple. To attend to the medical needs of a growing — and ageing — population you need more clinics and beds and wards and more doctors and nurses and other health professionals to staff those wards. And you need administrative staff to make sure all these things run properly. One doctor with 20 patients waiting to be seen who is unable to get off his phone to see even one patient does not cut it.

To do this requires A LOT OF MONEY to be invested. Sadly, governments of all political stripes have known this for the past 20 years and failed to lift more than their little fingers to address it.

It's not only the over-65 population that is increasing, but also the population at large. At the same time, modern medical treatment is becoming increasingly sophisticated — and expensive. In the 1990s if you had a stroke you were prescribed aspirin and hoped for the best. In the early 2000s a clot-busting drug became available that had to be administered within four and a half hours of the onset of symptoms. Strokes were now treated as emergencies.

In 2011 we began offering an emergency procedure called 'clot retrieval' to treat stroke. This is a procedure where the clot inside your brain gets sucked out using a wire sitting in your blood vessels. When I graduated from medical school the time window for this treatment was still four and a half hours. We had CT scans that could not always directly see whether a patient was having a stroke in that early phase, so there was a lot of educated guesswork. Sometimes we were wrong.

Since then we have acquired special CT scans that can pinpoint the exact location a stroke is occurring. The time window for clot retrieval has extended to 24 hours, meaning there are a lot more people getting emergency assessment and treatment for stroke.

Costs mount, old hospitals need replacing with modern, well-equipped facilities, yet the healthcare budget is not increasing sufficiently, and hasn't in decades.

Are the politicians making the right decisions?

We all have a say.

4.

HOSPITALS ARE FOR SICK PEOPLE

We were going through the list of patients on the medical ward at the start of the day.

'Then in Bed 14 we have Ms Jones. She's still waiting on that triple P and R paperwork to come through, then the family is going to start looking at residential facilities.'

A PPPR (Protection of Personal and Property Rights) is the long and complicated legal process by which a patient who is not able to make decisions for themself has a welfare guardian appointed to make decisions for them. While you are in good health you might appoint an enduring power of attorney (EPOA), who is activated if and when you lose your decision-making capacity. If you haven't done so, then things naturally get complicated.

'Right. So how much longer do we think that will take?' I asked.

'Dunno, but it's been 10 days already. Anyway, last night she spiked a fever and was started on nitrofurantoin [an antibiotic] for a positive urine.'

I breathed out heavily.

'Then next door we have Mr Smith. We've all agreed he needs rest-home placement; we just need to activate his EPOA. So he needs a capacity assessment.'

'Well, given that he thinks we're in Mexico and his neighbour across from him is selling tacos, I don't think that will take very long.'

The rest of the team chuckled.

'And he's still in Covid isolation until the 2nd.'

'You mean the Covid he got from hanging out in

hospital while he waited for something his family should have sorted out six months ago when he set the pantry alight?'

'Umm, yeah, I guess so,' my house officer said, looking down at his notes, apparently annoyed at my distracting comments when he just wanted to finish running through the list. 'He is due to finish Paxlovid today.'

I groaned. We were dishing out Paxlovid like candy.

'Right, then we have Mrs Brown in 21, who is also awaiting a rest-home placement. Her family went to visit one yesterday.'

'And?'

'Didn't like it. I think they're going to see another one today.'

'And what hospital-acquired infection does she have?'

'None yet,' my house officer remarked without a hint of irony.

'Is there anyone on this ward who actually has a medical problem?'

'Mrs Williams in 34. She's got pneumonia.'

'Ah yes, she was due for discharge today.'

'Well, no, that will be tomorrow now.'

'Why?'

'Family not available to pick her up till tomorrow.'

'Well, they'd better make themselves available. Either that or the ward clerk can order her a taxi.'

More chuckles.

'No, I'm frickin' serious,' I said. 'This is not a hotel. If she's medically ready for discharge, she goes. We have patients waiting in corridors and these people think this is the Intercontinental. And, as we all know, the longer they stay here, the more likely they are to contract a hospital-borne infection.'

I finished my long and weary ward round, during which I did not have to recall a single fact learnt in medical school. I walked down the long corridor lined with photos of smiling former patients, with speech bubbles added next to their comically oversized heads, filled with words of gratitude and thanks to the hospital. Some were designed to remind us of the hospital values we must always strive to uphold.

I recalled that during a recent online job application I had been asked to explain which of the organisation's values resonated most strongly with me.

'Empathy,' I wrote, unsure whether the arrow had hit the board or gone off into the crowd. It would have taken five seconds to google but that would have been five seconds of my life I would never get back. I got the job.

At the end of the corridor stood a skinny waist-high object that looked halfway between a podium and a music stand. On the flat surface on top were five buttons that ranged from green (with a happy face drawn on) to red (an angry face).

'Rate your experience with us!' a sign read.

I did what I did every time I walked down that corridor and tapped the red angry button. It made a beeping noise. That was probably the 26th time that week. I laughed as I walked past, finding unceasing amusement at the thought of somebody sitting in an office somewhere scratching their head over why patient satisfaction scores were so low in the annex corridor.

The doors to the stairwell creaked open. I let them go and, like a large juddering spring, they bounced back too far the other way, then back open before coming to rest. A wide beam of sunlight illuminated the dust hanging in the air. It bounced off the white walls and made me squint. Someone's footsteps echoed from above.

I walked slowly and deliberately up to the eighth floor. It was eerily quiet and the cellphone reception was poor here. It was one of only a few places you felt safe from the mayhem happening *out there*, if only for a minute or two.

I went into the registrar's office on the eighth floor. Two dusty computers with bulky monitors faced away from the window. Sundry medical journals and photocopied articles littered the bench, as did post-it notes with patient details scribbled on. The room was seldom used, but today Jenny was sitting at one of the computers, clacking away with a Word document open.

Jenny had practically finished her training and had a job as a gastrointestinal specialist lined up at the end of the month. She just had to make it through three more weeks in the trenches.

I sat down at the other computer. We nodded to each other and then sat in silence for a while.

Click. Clack clack clack. Click click.

I huffed and leaned my head back, holding my neck with my intertwined fingers and staring at the ceiling for a while.

'Hey Jenny, do you ever think we do more harm than good here?'

She regarded me intensely for a few seconds.

'Your week on the ward getting to you already?' She went back to clacking.

'I just . . . I just . . . I dunno.'

Another good lot of silence went by.

'A hospital is supposed to be a place where people come when they're unwell.'

'And you figured this out all by yourself? I'm so proud of you.'

Jenny's sarcasm was a way of trying to avoid a serious conversation.

'No, really. I saw 15 patients on the ward round today. Only one is in hospital because she was unwell. She's better now but still here. The rest are here cos they can't manage at home any longer. Literally 93 per cent of my ward round are waiting for a rest home, or a private hospital, or a dementia unit, or a home help package.'

'Sounds like an easy ward round.'

I tutted. Jenny stopped typing, placed her hands in her lap and turned around to face me.

'Look, I learnt a long time ago that the system is what it is,' she said. 'You can't change it. The work you train for isn't the job you end up doing. That's life.'

I made a face.

'At the end of the day, what else are you going to do?' she continued. 'Send them home so they can fall over or burn down the house?'

'Maybe.'

Jenny widened her eyes at me.

'Well, do you think that's less dangerous than detaining a bunch of vulnerable patients in this cesspool of infection and Covid?'

She shrugged. 'Detain is a strong word.'

'They *are* detained! None of them want to be here. Most of them don't have capacity to make their own decisions. I say that none of them are unwell, but actually many are — from infections they've caught from us. Half my ward round has had some kind of antibiotics in the last week. It's always the same story. They wait here for days and days until they spike a fever or their CRP [C-reactive protein, an inflammation marker] randomly starts climbing. And then we find they've got pneumonia, or a urinary tract infection, or Covid. Then their discharge gets further delayed because they're acutely "unwell".

'They sit for days and days. The physiotherapists and nurses are too overworked to mobilise them more than once a day, so they just lie in bed this whole time losing muscle. Then we get worried they're going to have a fall so we confine them to bed even more and they lose more muscle and get weaker, making them actually fall over.

'My grandpa looked like he was walking on a boat in a storm for the last 10 years of his life but he rarely fell over because he was in his house and he knew it well. The first thing he did when he was admitted to hospital was fall, due to being cooped up with other patients and being woken up a dozen times a night.

'Hell, one of our patients *died* over the weekend from hospital-acquired flu. I've got another who's been here so long and had so many complications of being an inpatient that, between you and me, nobody even remembers what she came to hospital for in the first place. Look me in the eye and tell me you really think that's safer than being at home.'

Jenny smiled in a way that said 'Oh, you sweet summer child.'

'I agree with everything you say. I also was once young and wanted to change everything. But . . .' She turned back to her screen. 'The world doesn't want to make sense and it never will, even long after you and I are gone, especially the world inside these walls. Everything involves some risk and uncertainty. But you know the first thing that happens when a patient falls over and breaks their hip in hospital? Your arse ends up in the news. Imagine if you send someone home and then they fall down the stairs. And the hospital won't protect you, they'll hang you out to dry.'

'That's why it needs to be a system-wide change. There needs to be funding for programmes to sort out all these placement issues in the community. Streamline taking care of people who are unsafe at home without cooping them up in here.'

'I'll tell you what, I'll give you the direct number for the prime minister, and you can discuss this directly.'

'All change starts somewhere!'

'And you need to start accepting the things you cannot change, Ivor.'

Clack clack.

◆◆◆

It was a long day. Not subjectively, although this was also true, but this is the name given to shifts that finish at 10 p.m., having started at 8 a.m.

I went to see my tenth patient of the day. The emergency department was particularly overwhelmed that day. You could barely find a computer or a space to sit on the flight deck (the central station overlooking all the rooms). Alarms were ringing out to starboard and going unattended. A psychotic patient was screaming out to port. To the aft, the charge nurse was pacing back and forth trying to have separate conversations on two phones at once.

I stood in the corner surveying the computers like a dog waiting for someone to look away so he can pounce at the food on the table. Someone left and I almost tripped over myself taking my opportunity. Mine now, sucker!

I began typing up the history of the patient I had just seen.

'2 months ago started having numb feet . . .'

'So why didn't you go to your GP about this?' I had asked him.

'My GP charges 90 bucks. I work 7 a.m. till 6 p.m. every day. I'd have to take a sick day to go to the doctor and wait 40 minutes. She spends 15 minutes with me, and half of that time she just types away on her computer without even looking at me.'

I raised an eyebrow.

'Yes, yes, I know what you're thinking, Doctor. You think I'm wasting your time.'

'No, no, of course not,' I said, lying through my teeth.

'Thing is, I woke up this morning and thought, what if this is something really serious? What if I have cancer?'

'You don't have cancer, which is the good news. The bad news is that your diabetes is not very well under control. You're starting to get nerve damage in your feet from high blood-sugar levels. We can't fix the damage that's already done, sadly, but it's really important we get that blood sugar much better controlled to stop this from getting worse.'

'Oh shit. Oh man, yeah, I mean, I'll be honest with you, Doc, I probably haven't been taking my meds as much as I should.'

Why would you ever think two months of tingly feet is an emergency? I thought to myself as I typed away, my loud tapping reflecting my frustration. Ultimately I was discharging this man back to the care of his GP anyway, so he would have to find a way to get around his issues with her bedside manner, or find a different GP.

Clearly the ad campaigns urging people to save the ED for *emergencies* were not having the desired effect.

My next patient was a man with shoulder pain.

I walked into the room. A stocky man was sitting up in the bed with his shirt off, while a worried-looking woman sat in the visitor's chair. He was quite sweaty, so that the ECG dots on his chest seemed to be slowly sliding off, like an ice-cream melting in the heat. All that stopped them from falling off completely was his thicket of chest hair.

'Hi there, I'm Ivor, one of the doctors on today. Nice to meet you.'

'Dan.'

He extended a clammy hand. Something felt off.

'Right, tell me about this shoulder, Dan.'

'Well, it's nothing much really. The left shoulder has been quite sore since this morning. I was not too fussed, to be honest. I was going to go in to work today and just work it off, but the missus insisted I come and get it checked out.'

His wife rolled her eyes.

A nurse poked her head through the curtain.

'Doctor, I have a fresh ECG for you. I think he's having a STEMI.'

I grabbed the ECG and looked at it, blinking a few times to make sure I wasn't imagining things.

'Umm, Dan, it looks like you're having a massive heart attack. We need to get you upstairs for an angiogram straight away.'

Upstairs in the angiography suite a cardiologist inserted a flexible wire through the blood vessel in his groin and snaked it all the way up to his heart. There they found a 100 per cent blockage of one of the main blood vessels supplying his heart, and placed a stent to open up the space.

Later, as I drove home, I reflected on the day. I felt embarrassed. I realised that day that patients have a right to seek help, and it's up to us to figure out whether it's an emergency or not. We can't expect patients to do their own triage. We are blazing hypocrites, really. On the one hand we run ad campaigns showing people clutching their chests, saying: 'If you have any concern, call an ambulance straight away,' while on the other hand we tell people to diagnose themselves before presenting to the ED.

It is too easy to become judgemental.

The reality is that it's not patients coming to the ED for non-emergencies who crowd the corridors. They may soak up emergency doctors' time and fill up the waiting room, but ultimately they are discharged. They don't contribute to bed-block.

And actually they are making a rational economic choice. A $90 fee is a lot of money, and if you work all the hours your GP's surgery is open, it's a pretty straightforward decision. The ED is open at nights and weekends, and it's free. The issue of non-emergency patients in the ED is the symptom of a wider problem with healthcare.

As anyone who has tried to make a GP appointment lately knows, there are not enough GPs to take care of our growing and increasingly sick population. Although primary care is government-subsidised, GP practices are expected to run like a business. Mix an unmet demand with a requirement to stay financially viable and the resulting fees and unavailability push more and more patients away from primary care.

How can this problem be solved? I don't work in primary care but some of my friends do, and they have some ideas.

First up, the funding model needs rethinking. Public funding of GPs is based on the number of enrolled patients, so-called capitation rates, rather than how often the patients are seen or the complexity of their health issue/s. GPs need to be funded for the work they actually do, including all the admin that goes along with every appointment.

For every chunk of time actually spent seeing a patient, another decent chunk is spent sending referral letters, following up test results and communicating them to patients, reading letters from hospital appointments and actioning the instructions, refilling prescriptions remotely, answering patient emails and filling out ACC forms. They are not actually paid directly for doing this, so a lot of this work happens after hours or during lunch breaks.

GPs cut back their hours so as to not fall apart at the seams, and this only puts more pressure on the workforce. In the meantime, the proportion of doctors who are GPs has fallen by 10 per cent since the turn of the millennium.

GPs in training are paid peanuts compared with their colleagues in hospital specialties, which doesn't help GP recruitment.

They also have the absolute hardest job. By the time a patient makes their way to my guardianship in the ICU, it is very clear that they are sick. They have had a battery of tests run, which I am free to peruse at my leisure, and they have skilled nurses to watch over them 24/7.

In contrast, nine out of ten patients who turn up to

see their GP with a *new* problem have nothing wrong with them that can't be fixed with either time, exercise or paracetamol (although many GP appointments are for old, chronic and complex problems). It is the job of the GP to identify the tenth patient, the one who has some nasty, saliva-drooling, fang-bearing, beast of a disease lying in wait in the shrubbery, who is disguised as one of the other nine. Which of these babies with a snotty nose in winter has meningitis; which is the needle in the haystack of common colds?

Most of the reason why people end up in hospital is complications of chronic conditions that have got out of control. Diabetes, high blood pressure, high cholesterol, smoking and obesity are the reason our hospitals are full. They lead to heart attacks, strokes, kidney failure, blockages of arteries, lung disease, and skin and lung infections. As well as being problems by themselves, all these things make a person frail, so they are more likely to fall over and break a bone. Managing all of these things is the bread and butter of GPs, so the return on investing in primary care is enormous. One good GP can do more good than ten intensive care doctors.

Maybe one of the reasons primary care is under-resourced is the increasing trend of super-specialisation. More money is being spent on the fringes of medicine. We throw cash at fancy robotic surgery and machines in the ICU that keep people alive forever. Shiny things look good, but we lack evidence that this is money well spent, in terms of the overall health of the population. Student doctors see the dollars flowing into super-specialised areas of medicine, and not into the areas that we know for sure make a difference. It is no surprise that they are not flocking to GP training.

So when you can't provide good services or good access to help and residential care in the community, the hospitals fill up, the beds become blocked, and everybody gets mad at the emergency department, who are blameless. The ED waiting room is further engorged by patients unable to access their GPs. This is why every so often you see a story in the news about someone who died after spending all day in the waiting room.

It all comes down to money in the end. There is no free lunch, I'm afraid.

5.

PUBLIC, PRIVATE & PROFIT

New Zealand's private health system offers those with means the ability to buy the services of a specialist rather than wait weeks or months to be seen in the public system — usually by the same specialists. These specialists generally split their time between the public system (public hospitals) and private practice, which is more lucrative.

For six months I was a relief registrar. This meant that whenever a registrar was off sick or on leave, I covered the gap. One week I was doing cardiology consults. I would see any patient referred by the general teams who had a cardiac problem that needed specialist input, and discuss them with the cardiologist on call. Given the popular modern diet of fat and sugar, this was one the busier jobs in the hospital.

Mrs Taylor was 66 years old and had been having dizzy spells for the past year. The day before she had blacked out and whacked her arm in the fall, breaking her humerus. She'd done a good job, too. The fracture was reasonably displaced, meaning that the two ends of the fracture did not line up well.

I was bending over listening to her heart with my stethoscope. I'd seen the results of that morning's echocardiogram, so it was a surprise that it all sounded very normal. Clearly the narrowing was so severe that no abnormal sound could actually come through.

'Lub-dub. Lub-dub,' with every heartbeat.

I stood back up and rearranged the front of her hospital gown. The front and back were joined by buttons sitting across the shoulders. I got to the last one before I realised I'd got them out of synch and had to start over.

'Well, Doc, what's going on you reckon? My GP tried to get them to do a scan of my heart to figure it out, but I'm still on the waiting list after eight months!'

'You've got a severe narrowing of the valve that allows blood to pass from your heart to the rest of your body. This makes it hard for the heart to push out as much blood as it needs to, and if your brain doesn't get enough blood you black out,' I explained.

'Wow. Jeez. I knew something was up with my ticker. So if I'd had my heart scan earlier, rather than waiting till I fell, I wouldn't have broken my arm.'

I frowned empathetically. She looked down at the ground and heaved a big sigh.

'Why couldn't they get me in sooner then?'

'Your situation is not unusual, sadly. I've had patients who've had to wait for over a year.'

'Well, it's just not right, not right at all.'

She looked off into the distance a while longer.

'Well, no use crying over spilt milk, I guess. What now then?'

'Well, your broken arm makes it quite complicated. The usual treatment for a normally healthy person is open heart surgery to replace the valve. But this broken arm of yours probably needs an operation before that, and putting you under anaesthesia with a severely narrowed aortic valve is very dangerous. So it's kind of a Catch-22.'

I paused to make sure she had processed all this before continuing.

'It might be that we need to do a minimally invasive type of procedure to replace the valve first. Then we can go on to fix the arm. Or it may be that we have the option of treating the arm without surgery, but we need to discuss that with the bone doctors.'

She nodded slowly.

'That's a lot of information I've thrown at you. Any questions?'

She shook her head.

'In short, the situation is quite complex and the specialists need to discuss it and decide on the best thing to do. We'll chat with you some more soon. In the meantime you'll also need to have an angiogram to make sure there are no blockages of your heart arteries.'

'Okay, thanks Doc.'

She looked deflated as I walked out of the room and towards the central station to pick up the next patient's folder.

I introduced myself to the patient in the room next to Mrs Taylor.

'So, it says here you've been recently diagnosed with SVT, but we can't find anything in your records about it.'

SVT stands for supraventricular tachycardia, an arrhythmia starting from the top chambers of the heart that makes the heartbeat extremely fast. It comes in episodes.

'Oh, yeah, no, I've been seeing a cardiologist privately.'

Of course she had. She's probably had a million-dollar work-up and none of it available to see on our computer system.

'He put me on a beta-blocker,' she continued. 'It's been working well, but I've had a couple of attacks leading up to the big one yesterday.'

'Have you ever had an echocardiogram?'

Ms Lyell chuckled.

'Oh yes, of course. He's done an echo, and I've had a CT angiogram as well. That was all normal. He did a treadmill test as well — I have a copy of that somewhere if you need it. A Holter monitor too, but we didn't manage to catch any episodes.'

'And how long ago did you do all this?'

'I saw him about three months ago.'

Noticing me standing with mouth agape, she raised her eyebrows and leaned forward, clutching the collar of her gown.

'Something wrong, dear?'

'No, no, not at all. I'm just impressed at how thorough your cardiologist has been.'

I paused for a second.

'It's very good you've managed to get all this done privately. Getting all those tests in the public system would take . . . well, somewhere between 10 and 150 years.'

She chortled.

'Yes, I know. I'm very glad I have health insurance.'

I proceeded with my examination.

I had seen seven patients that morning and needed to

contact the on-call cardiologist to discuss them and make sure they agreed with my plans. The referring teams were not really interested in my opinion; I was a nobody. They wanted the specialist's opinion. I was just the go-between.

I strode briskly, trying to contain the bristling sensation that was building up under my skin. I pondered how the cardiologist would respond if this was Ms Lyell's first presentation with SVT and I had suggested doing all those tests in the public system. They would probably laugh at me and hang up the phone. She'd be lucky to even get half of those tests done.

It's just so fucking unfair.

Specialists like to wax philosophical to junior doctors about relying on your clinical skills rather than ordering tests. Until they stand to profit from such tests. Funny how clinical judgement can change depending on incentives.

What made the situation even more bullshit was that her hospital neighbour had suffered a badly broken arm because she couldn't access a simple test like an echocardiogram in the public system.

I was getting exercised about it all, so once I got to the doctors' office I took a minute to take some deep breaths before calling the on-call specialist.

'Hey, it's Ivor here. I've seen a bunch of patients this morning and need to discuss them with you.'

'I'm in private this morning. Can you call back after lunch?'

◆◆◆

Many years later my ICU colleagues and I were sitting around the tea-room couches, sipping coffee. The couches were dilapidated and you didn't want to spend too much time thinking about when they had last been cleaned. Actually, that was true of anything in this place.

I had just finished recounting this story.

'That is such bullshit!' exclaimed Vicky. 'It's double-dipping. They're on call in the public system and running their private clinic at the same time!'

The group murmured in agreement.

'The hospital needs to crack down on this kind of stuff,' she continued.

The grey-haired doctor with the thousand-yard stare sitting on the only armchair cleared his throat. Everybody turned to listen.

'Yeah, except if you do that, they all just fuck off to private permanently, and leave the public system even more fucked. These guys can basically do whatever they like because they always have that threat available.'

Everybody stared at the ground and sipped contemplatively.

John continued. 'You know that's why we get paid so unevenly in public. The specialists who have the option of doing private work get paid more to keep them working in public.'

'Yeah, and they get the private work after they've made a name for themselves in public,' said Vicky. 'That new guy we met the other day who's just qualified — what's his name? Anyway, he'll float around the public system for a couple of years, get his name on a bunch of clinic letters, GPs will start recognising his name, see him as someone to be trusted, someone to refer to, then bang! He's outta here.'

She leaned back and took a big swig from her cup.

I stared off into the distance and wondered whether maybe we were all just jealous. The ICU did not offer much option for private work, so maybe we were all just mad at our own choices.

While everyone chatted away I thought back to the first time I had met John. It was four years earlier when I was a registrar on rotation. It was the middle of winter. Rain was battering the few bits of glass that you could usually rely on to let in some light. It was a good metaphor for the state of the hospital. My emergency pager had not stopped all day. I had contemplated walking up to the roof and throwing it over, but I didn't want to get wet.

I had been asked to review a patient on the surgical ward who was 'struggling to oxygenate well' and might need to be transferred to the ICU.

The intensive care unit takes care of patients who need machines or infusions to keep them alive. The most common reason is that the oxygen level in their blood is low, and they need high amounts of oxygen, or even a breathing tube and a ventilator.

I read the patient's notes: 54-year-old male, admitted a week earlier with pancreatitis. Recent blood tests indicated his condition was getting worse, and his oxygen levels were slowly falling.

When the pancreas gets badly inflamed, fluid builds up around it and inside the abdominal cavity, the same way your ankle swells up when you twist it. This swelling pushes up on the lungs and can shrink them. The fluid can also make its way into the chest cavity.

Their notes often belie how the patient actually looks. I always feel a fluttering in the stomach in the 10 seconds between reading the notes and stepping into the patient's room, unsure whether I will see someone who, all things considered, doesn't look too bad, or whether I am walking into a disaster. Interpreting the way a patient 'looks' comes down to instinct, built up over years of experience, the same way you recognise a dark alleyway as being dangerous without having to articulate the exact reasons why.

My first thought when I cast my eyes on this patient was: 'This guy is *sick*.' My second thought was: 'Where the hell is everybody?'

When I say *sick*, I don't mean the way you might look when you have the flu — washed out and tired, with baggy eyes and a runny nose. 'Sick' in medical language means the person is going to die in the next few hours if you don't do something. Our man with pancreatitis had a glazed look in his eyes. The corners of his mouth were turned down. He looked grey and shiny with sweat. He was taking rapid, shallow breaths and the muscles on his neck were bulging with every breath.

I stepped out and called John, who was the on-call consultant. 'He looks bad,' I said. 'He needs to be intubated.'

I heard swearing on the other end of the line. Then: 'Okay, okay, I'll be right up.'

Intubating is the process of sending someone off to sleep and inserting a plastic breathing tube into their windpipe.

After seeing the patient for himself, John agreed with me. 'I think we have time to take him down to the unit and do it there.'

He paused for a moment and stroked his grey goatee.

'Do you know when this patient was last seen by a surgical specialist?'

'Pass.'

'Come with me.'

He grabbed me by the arm and dragged me to a nearby desk before I could protest. I stood next to him while he flicked through pages of medical notes, like a child waiting for their father to finish work so they could go and play.

'Here!'

He jabbed his finger down hard on the paper, partially scrunching the page.

'The 25th! The fucking 25th! That was the last time he was seen by a specialist. On the day of admission. What day is it today?'

'The 31st,' I offered timidly.

'That's right. Six days. This patient has been on this ward circling the drain for six days, and has not been seen by a specialist once in that time.' The vein in his forehead was starting to bulge.

'You know why that is, right? You know what the problem is, don't you?'

I stared back at him with wide eyes and slowly shook my head.

He turned to a computer and started typing furiously. He opened a website and, before it had even loaded, stood up sharply, inadvertently propelling the swivel chair backwards with such force that it narrowly missed a group of startled nurses before crashing into a nearby supply cupboard.

'*That's* the problem!'

He walked away.

I looked at the screen. It was a picture of the surgeon in question, with a beaming smile plastered on their face. Underneath were the words: 'Generic-Feel-Good-Clinic-Name, where we provide you with friendly and holistic surgical care.' It was the website for their private practice.

◆◆◆

Once you finish your first two years of post-medical-school rotations around different specialties as a house officer, you can apply to a training programme in the specialty in which you want to spend the rest of your life working.

The public have the idea that there are general practitioners and specialists, but this is not true. Every senior doctor is a specialist. GPs are specialists in general practice, and work in primary care rather than hospitals.

The specialist training programmes are run by joint New Zealand–Australia colleges, and all training is in the public system. Some programmes, such as intensive care, where I am about to finish training in mid-2025, are not very competitive because who wants to spend the rest of their life sleeping in the hospital at night? Others require a superhuman CV to get into.

I had known Hohepa since we were lab partners during first-year biomedical science, both aiming to get accepted to medical school. The first words he ever said to me were, 'Hey, I'm Hohepa.'

The second were: 'I want to be a neurosurgeon.'

This man was on a mission from day one. He always wore nice pointy-toe shoes with such a shine that you almost had to wear sunglasses around him. You could hear him coming around the corner from the clacking they made on the linoleum.

The tutor who marked our lab assignments was, like me, from the former Yugoslavia. Every time we had lab, Hohepa would feign interest and ask him how his PhD was going, what project he was working on, how life was going, all of which drew gushing responses.

We somehow ended up with pretty good grades on our lab assignments, despite managing to burn the electrical cord on the Bunsen burner more than once. One assignment involved synthesising some kind of crystals.

'Hey, Ivor,' Hohepa began, with the kind of inflection that told me I needed to pay attention.

'Yeah?'

'We get marked on the quantity of crystals we produce, right?'

'Yeah,' I said, with growing excitement about where this was going.

'Well, if we just triple the quantity of the reactants, we should get triple the quantity of crystals, right?'

'Hohepa, time and time again you end up pulling through for me, man. You're a fucking genius.'

Fifteen years on, I regularly run into Hohepa at work. On one of these occasions we were standing in the coffee queue chatting about life. I noticed his shoes were dull and his scrubs crumpled. He kept yawning and rubbing his eyes.

'When do the applications for neurosurgery open?' I asked.

'Next month,' he replied. 'But I'm not going to apply this year.'

My jaw dropped. 'What do you mean? Why not?'

'My application just isn't strong enough, you know? I want to give myself more time to buff up the CV, not waste an attempt, then come in strong next year with a better chance of getting on.'

'Dude, you have a PhD. A PhD in brain stuff. What more could they want?'

He grinned wistfully.

'Well, unfortunately so do a lot of others.'

'So what do they have that you don't? Friends in high places?'

He laughed.

On average, only about a third of applicants to surgical programmes are accepted each year. In some years and in some specialties this has been as low as one-sixth. The pool of applicants includes Australia, and neurosurgery, paediatric surgery and cardiac surgery have sometimes gone for years without selecting a single Kiwi applicant.

The surgical specialties are the worst, but practically every specialty has more applications than training positions available. Other competitive specialties include radiology, anaesthesia, cardiology, gastroenterology, ophthalmology and dermatology.

So is it the case that these specialties are just incredibly popular, with more applicants than are needed? Why would they be so popular? The common denominator, if you look at the list above, is that those specialties offer the most scope for private work. They are 'procedure-based', and procedures reimburse well.

But while this is a factor, we also know there are shortages in the public system of every single type of specialist, and this shortage is only predicted to widen over the coming years as the needs of the health sector grow. So we need to train more specialists of every type. Why is this not happening?

Both left- and right-wing governments have publicly acknowledged the need to train more doctors, and have pledged to increase medical school numbers. Without increasing the number of jobs for them when they graduate, however, creating extra places at medical school will do about as much to fix the doctor shortage as putting up tents on Parliament's lawn will do to fix the housing crisis. For at least a decade we have been graduating more first-year doctors than there are jobs for them.

The problem occurs at the point where you take junior doctors and train them to be specialists, and this part is not fully within the government's control. The number of training spots offered each year is determined by the Australasian specialist medical colleges, and by the number of government-funded training spots. The exact process by which it all occurs is a bit muddy, but the colleges decide on each year's intake.

Could it be that the colleges are trying to artificially restrict training places because they know that a shortage of specialists keeps them with their hands at the private market's throat? I'm not the first one to voice such a crazy idea — colleges have been investigated for anti-competitive practices by both the New Zealand Commerce Commission and its Australian counterpart. No confirmation of wrongdoing has ever been found, but why would it? It's unlikely anyone's keeping minutes. Those colleges hold the power and their specialist members have strong incentives to keep their numbers tight.

◆◆◆

A compulsory part of my training was spending a year doing anaesthesia. Sending people off to sleep for an operation is much like what I hear about being a pilot: 99 per cent routine and 1 per cent sheer terror. You do your takeoff and landing (putting the patient to sleep and waking them up at the end), and in between there is a lot of sitting around, staying vigilant, and trying to pick up on small problems before they become big problems. There is also a lot of time to do Wordle, or Sudoku, or manage your sharemarket portfolio if you have one. You're also a fly on the wall to a lot of interesting conversations between surgeons.

One particularly complex orthopaedic operation had three surgeons scrubbed in. I was doing my best to appear fascinated by the dotted green blips that punctuated the monitor screen while all my attention was actually focused on the conversation taking place on the other side of the drape, muffled by the surgeons' masks. They were discussing the current pool of junior doctors.

'Oh yeah, no, he's definitely getting on this year.'

'Yeah, solid worker, great CV. I've given him a great reference.'

'Did you hear BJ is applying again?'

'Ha! That joker is never getting on. Dunno why he keeps trying. Surely he knows.'

'Well, has anyone told him?'

The sound of metal on metal pierced the air as they drove a large nail into the patient's bone.

'I just hope they keep the numbers similar to last year.'

'Yup, there's been a lot of new trainees coming through recently. Gotta protect the patch!'

◆◆◆

Some applicants' fates are likely decided well before the formal process begins. Medicine is a small world, and in a small world a lot depends on who you know and whether they like you. There are many very capable doctors who managed to piss off the wrong person and will probably never get onto specialist training. They and others who can't build an impressive-enough CV usually work for years as 'non-training' registrars until the exploitation gets too much and they give up on their dream, to pursue a different specialty or quit medicine altogether. Some specialists don't mind having experienced hands working for them when they are on call, even if they know those same hands are not getting anything out of the deal.

◆◆◆

Now, however, I will finish this chapter with a story that illustrates my own hypocrisy.

My wife went to a dermatology associate (like GPs but with extra training in skin conditions) because she was losing a patch of hair on the front of her scalp. A previous doctor had injected the forehead with steroids to help hair regrowth. A couple of months later she noticed a bony growth in the same spot.

The dermatology associate we saw was very experienced and well-read and told us that this might be coup de sabre, a rare autoimmune condition that destroys the tissues in the scalp, including bone. Without a strong immune-suppressing medication it would progress. But alternatively, it might just be skin atrophy (thinning) as a side-effect of the steroid shot. In this case it would get better by itself with time. A biopsy of the scalp would tell us.

My wife was understandably freaked out. I had never heard of coup de sabre but I explained that skin atrophy after a steroid shot occurred in at least one in a hundred cases, probably more. By contrast, the number of people who had the autoimmune condition was one in a million, from what I could find on Google. Almost certainly the biopsy would show that it was all fine.

We had the biopsy booked in for a week later. Even though this was all being done privately, the sample would be analysed in a public lab. As usual, the lab had a huge backlog, so it would take some weeks for the result to come back.

My wife stared at the floor and shook her head.

'No, I can't wait that long. I need to know sooner.'

While I realised that our situation wasn't as bad as some poor sod waiting on a cancer diagnosis, at that point I didn't really give a shit about anybody else's plight.

'Surely there is a way we can get it faster?' I said, attempting my best assertive-but-not-too-pushy tone.

The doctor looked at me sideways.

'Well, there is a private lab we can get it sent to and it'll be done by Monday. But you guys don't have insurance, right? It costs $300.'

'We'll pay.'

I went to work on Monday, waiting all morning for the call that would take the tension out of my shoulders, the call to say it was all fine and we could stop worrying. Normal life could resume.

I came out of a patient's room and saw I had missed a call from my wife. I almost vomited out my jumping heart. I found a private room and called her back, but my hands were shaking so much I could barely hold the phone to my ear.

Her voice was like a mouse. I knew what this meant.

'Ivor, it's not good. The biopsy shows the bad one.'

All sound and vision went fuzzy for a few seconds. My fingertips felt ice-cold. I opened and closed my mouth a few times, but nothing came out.

'Ivor?'

I had no choice but to find some strength. I took some deep breaths.

'It's okay, baby, it's okay. I know this is not the news we wanted, but it's what we've been dealt, and . . . we'll find a way to get through it. We have no choice. Why don't I come home and let's . . . let's just sit with this for a bit, and then figure out a way forward, one step at a time.'

I found someone to cover the rest of my shift and went home.

On the way I could feel the skin just above my collar bones bouncing up and down from my heartbeat. I started thinking about what measures I needed to put in place. Now that she had to be on immunosuppressants I was going to have to go back to wearing a mask at work. I was going to have to be careful to separate my work clothes from my home clothes. Probably come home and shower straight away before kissing her hi. Did she need to be on preventative antibiotics? I texted my friend who was an infectious diseases specialist.

We wanted children and were looking to get pregnant in the next few years, but she couldn't get pregnant while she was taking immunosuppressants. And she would be on them for years.

For the first time, I used my connections. I emailed someone I had worked with a long time ago who now worked at a fertility clinic. She still remembered me. She got us an appointment the following week, and by the end of that week we were all ready to go with egg freezing. We'd done the education session, we'd read the booklets; all we had to do was book a time to start the injections that would make her ovaries go crazy and produce a year's worth of eggs in one go. These would then be collected and saved for the future.

'So, since I'm infertile and this situation is out of our control, hopefully the treatment will be funded?' My wife raised her eyebrows and turned her head sideways.

The obstetrician smiled sympathetically.

'Well, the unfortunate news is that it won't. The meds don't actually make you infertile, as once you stop taking them your fertility returns to normal.'

'But I can't stop the medication for a long time.' She half-smiled, half-frowned.

'I know, it sucks,' the doctor said.

We fell silent.

It would add up to $16,000 — a small fortune. Fuck it, I thought. That's why you put away money for a rainy day.

The obstetrician had such a sweet manner, it made everything seem not quite as bad. I wondered whether she remembered me. Over a decade ago she had been the obstetric registrar when I was a medical student on placement. She sent me to put an IV line in a pregnant patient. Pregnant patients have massive veins; the phrase is that you could drive a truck through them. But I had to trudge back half an hour later to report that I had tried three times and failed. She had scoffed and looked at me in disgust. I pondered now that even nice people can come across mean in some environments.

The dermatology associate wanted my wife to consult a specialist dermatologist and a rheumatologist (a specialist in autoimmune disorders). This was a complex and rare condition, outside of her comfort zone.

Thankfully she had been on a waiting list to see a dermatologist from when she first noticed the problem. She eventually got in to see him after four months of waiting. Damn public system, right? No, this was four months on a *private* waiting list. The waiting time for public? Not even the devil really knew. The public wait time for a rheumatologist was the same. The rheumatologist was going to be the key player, because, even though it was a rare disease, they knew the most about it.

She was advised the best thing to do was to harvest her eggs, then start on the medication straight after, while waiting for a rheumatology appointment. We booked in for the 'egg injections'.

I was in denial. The odds were so astronomically small that she would have this really rare disease over a very common one. Why did she have to be the one in a million? I became obsessed with the idea that the biopsy was wrong. I got into such a state that I could feel the cogs in my head turning every waking moment. I forgot what it was like to feel tired. Eating, drinking and showering became obstacles. Any human interaction irritated me.

I started to fantasise about how life had felt before we knew anything about this stupid condition. How pleasurable it would be sitting in the car in traffic, or pushing a shopping cart through the mall — doing the ordinary everyday things we did before we knew. I bargained that if this would all just disappear, we would never wish for anything ever again. I convinced myself that if I thought this hard enough, it would be so.

Outside of work and sleep, all my energy was focused on researching this condition, its appearances on biopsy, what steroid atrophy looked like on biopsy, and whether there was any chance the two could be confused. I read case report after case report. I emailed private laboratories around the globe asking for a second opinion. I checked my email every hour, and as the days went by without a single reply, I became more and more angry at my powerlessness. The world had dealt its shattering blow, and then just moved on. We were the victims of a providential hit and run.

The world had played dirty, so I felt justified in playing dirty back. I hated people who abused their connections to get ahead. Now I was going to become the very thing I hated. I didn't care. I felt no guilt. Everything is different when it's personal.

I told my wife to hold off starting the meds until I got her a private appointment with the best rheumatologist in town. I had never met him, but I used my work email. He offered us a spot the following week, even though I knew his waiting list was longer than that. The medical community looks after its own. 'Professional courtesy', they call it.

He examined my wife meticulously, took her history and read the biopsy report.

'I think this is steroid-induced fat atrophy. Your skin doesn't feel tight and scarred the way it would if it was something serious. This will get better by itself over the next six months.'

My wife burst into tears. I stared at the floor and let out a chuckle. With the breath that escaped my mouth went the horrible concoction of fear, anger and tiredness that had contaminated me for the past couple of months. The buzzing sound inside my head faded instantly. All I wanted to do was sit in that chair and enjoy the moment.

After wiping away her tears, my wife asked the obvious question.

'What about the biopsy? Was it wrong?'

'Well, no it wasn't, but it wasn't right either. A biopsy just shows you what the tissue looks like. Sometimes that's enough on its own to make a diagnosis, like with cancer. Most of the time though, that doesn't make a diagnosis. What makes a diagnosis is having the right appearance on the biopsy under the right clinical context. This is the wrong context.'

He looked at me as if to say, 'You know what I'm talking about.'

As we drove home I thought about how unfair it all was. Not for us. Not for people who had connections, who had the knowledge, and who had the means to afford private healthcare. But for the average Kiwi in our situation, who might have ended up spending years on powerful meds for a condition they didn't have, unable to have babies, and still waiting for a specialist appointment.

Healthcare in the private system is no better than in public, but it is faster because it is not accessible to all. Even for the exclusive few it leaves a lot to be desired. One system cannot pick up the slack for the other. It is mostly all the same doctors manning both. You cannot feed private, and expand its role, without starving public, because there are no specialists sitting around in want of work. Nor are the two systems designed to overlap neatly; when private patients have major complications, they are transferred to the public system, which has the appropriate infrastructure to deal with more acute problems. If everybody in the country had health insurance, private care would be oversubscribed just like the failing public system. Healthcare is a zero-sum game.

My wife's hair and forehead are back to normal.

6.

THE TEST IS NOT THE DISEASE

You may find it difficult to accept that a doctor's hands could be more reliable than a biopsy. But that's the wrong way to think about it.

Some years ago I was walking across the canteen in the evening, spilling chicken noodle broth over my scrubs. As junior doctors we got free food in the canteen, but today the menu was uninspiring. There being a regular 'fish'n'chip Friday', it was suspicious when the same meal was on offer on Saturday. And every so often it was nice to treat yourself to Uber Eats.

It had been a sleepy kind of day. Rain gently pattered on the windows, and the corridors were filled with a thick humid smell. A few visitors were scattered across the large central atrium, speaking softly to each other. All I could hear was the sound of water droplets on metal and the occasional ring of the front-desk landline. I felt as if I was walking through some desolate marshland on my way to dinner. It was hard not to think that half the city had gone away for the long weekend.

Things had an unnatural ease to them. I was carrying the emergency pager and it had barely gone off all day. All the patients seemed to be getting better. The staffroom cutlery drawer actually had clean forks and the fax machine had not broken down all day.

I had spent the last half-hour exploring a maintenance corridor on the lower ground floor. My head hairs just avoided scratching the roof, and large metal pipes lined the corridor on the right-hand side. Every 20 metres or so I came across an abandoned child's cot. Sealed-off doorways branching from the corridor were plastered with signs that read: 'Danger. Do not open. Asbestos risk.' I could feel the goosebumps rising.

Days like this were rare, and when they did happen you almost started to wish for some work because you could feel the rust building up in your brain. But you also knew it wouldn't last. That knowledge was enough to stop you from eating your meal in slow, deliberate bites. Instead, you scarfed it down just as you would on any other day.

True to form, I was barely halfway through my dinner when the pager went off. An emergency on one of the surgical wards. Emergencies only ever happen when you sit down to eat, or sit down on the toilet, or when you're embroiled in another emergency.

The first rule in an emergency is to take your own pulse. Nobody tears along the corridors knocking people out of the way like they do on TV. If you turn up to the patient sweaty and flustered, you're no good to anyone.

The patient was an elderly gentleman who had had an operation to remove cancer from his oesophagus [food pipe]. The operation is called an Ivor Lewis. Essentially it involves cutting out a whole section of the oesophagus, so you are left with a piece of the pipe at either end, and these two have to be stitched back together. The site where these two ends are joined is called an anastomosis.

The tissues in the oesophagus are very fragile, and one of the main complications of this surgery is a leak at the site of the anastomosis — even a tiny gap in the stitching could allow fluid to leak out and cause infection.

This is not because the surgeon did a bad job; it's because stitching together a food pipe is not quite the same as doing embroidery, and it's impossible to achieve perfection.

The man was sitting bolt upright gasping for air. An oxygen monitor was struggling to get a reading. Every so often it beeped and showed 82 per cent. Meanwhile a confused flight of activity was happening around him. One nurse was applying oxygen. Another was taking his blood pressure and writing down the numbers. A third nurse was flushing some kind of medication through his IV line.

A house officer stood nearby looking around aimlessly, eyes darting back and forth as he tried to find some way of being helpful. He tried to question one of the nurses but she was too preoccupied. The emergency outreach nurse was talking to another nurse who seemed to know the most about the patient, trying to get a handover. Another house officer was talking to the surgical registrar who had just appeared, and giving her the exact same handover. The patient added to the din by yelping as yet another house officer knelt down by his side and was fishing around in his wrist to get a blood sample.

Everyone was well trained and doing the right thing, but in an emergency what matters is everyone doing the right thing at the same time. Managing the team is as important as managing the patient.

I took a breath and yelled over the din.

'Oi!!!'

Everyone stopped and looked.

'Okay, my name's Ivor and I'll be team-leading this code. Could everyone else quickly introduce themselves?'

We did a quick circuit around the room.

'Right, now could someone who knows the patient please summarise for everyone else what is going on.'

The surgical registrar cleared her throat and stepped forward.

'Okay, Wiremu is 68. He had an Ivor Lewis 72 hours ago which was uncomplicated, he stepped down to the ward yesterday, but this afternoon he's deteriorated with fever, tachypnoea [abnormally rapid breathing] and hypoxia [low oxygen levels]. His blood pressure and heart rate are okay. He had an X-ray about 30 minutes ago which showed some atelectasis [lung collapse] at his left base, but nothing else notable.'

The jumble was starting to disentangle itself.

'Okay,' I said, 'so I think Wiremu needs intubating. Our priority at the moment is to try to stabilise his oxygen levels enough that we can transfer him to the ICU rather than having to do it here on the ward. Let's get the Hudson mask on him and see how he goes with that; we won't be able to transfer him with the high flow he has at the moment. Anyone have any other ideas about what needs to be done?'

'He has some history of heart failure,' one of the nurses chipped in. 'He normally takes furosemide [a diuretic] but it hasn't been prescribed on the ward. Should we give him some?'

'Sounds like an excellent idea. Give him 40 milligrams IV.'

After we stabilised Wiremu's oxygen levels he needed a CT scan to look for a leak from the oesophagus. It was best to do it while he was still awake and before we intubated him so he could swallow some contrast liquid that would make the scan more accurate. But given how fragile his breathing was, I worried that he might not tolerate lying flat in the CT scanner. And yet if we intubated him first, it was going to be impossible to give him the contrast. A rock and a hard place.

No textbook prepares you for these scenarios or tells you the right answer. You just have to make the best decision you can. You may never know if it was the right one.

We decided we would try for the scan first, our eyes glued to his oxygen levels the whole time. It would only take a minute or two. His oxygen levels dipped to 90 per cent but he got through okay and we transferred him to the ICU.

The CT scan showed no leak.

The next morning Wiremu was worse. His X-ray showed half of the left lung was filled with fluid.

The intensive care specialist for the day stood around sipping his morning coffee.

'So, Ivor, what do you want to do with this patient?'

Put on the spot, I opened my mouth, then closed it, then opened it again.

'Um, well . . . I suppose we should make sure he's on

some antibiotics . . . and . . . ultrasound his chest and see if we can drain the fluid.'

'Okaaay,' he said in a drawn-out way, 'why do you think this patient developed a pleural effusion [fluid around the lung] overnight?'

'Most likely it's infection?' I ended the sentence with an upward inflection.

The toying smile on the specialist's face disappeared.

'Ivor, what about a leak?'

'But he had a scan yesterday that didn't show any leak.'

'No, it didn't show any leak. Does that mean he's not leaking?'

'I don't understand.'

He shook his head.

'Ivor, my boy, that was a CT scan. It was *not* the patient. The patient is the one with the disease, not the CT machine. The test is not the disease. What is the leak rate for an Ivor Lewis?'

'High. About 30 per cent.'

'Great. And what is the most likely reason for a patient to crap out three days after their Ivor Lewis with fluid seeping into their chest cavity?'

'A leak?'

Wiremu was sent for a repeat CT. It showed a massive leak.

◆◆◆

We live in a time of fancy machines and technology. It is tempting to think that we will eventually reach the point where they tell us everything we need to know, but I don't believe this will ever happen.

Medicine uses a way of thinking that is completely alien to most people. Our thinking has to be based on probability, because unless you walk into the ED with a sword sticking into your abdomen, it is hard for a doctor to be 100 per cent sure about what is wrong with you. The body never gives us perfect feedback. It is not like working in other industries, where you can judge the success of something by whether it functions or sells. In medicine it is hard to even know a lot of the time whether the treatment you prescribe is actually helping the patient, because human bodies have this annoying habit of being able to heal themselves.

We can only ever estimate what is going on, based on probability, then try to shift that probability as close as we can to 100 per cent while never reaching it. The information we get about a patient from our eyes and ears sets most of that probability. Medical testing only shifts the probability by small degrees either way.

Let's say you're cooking some chicken. You want to know if it is safe to eat. You know that chicken is supposed to be cooked to 75°C, and you have a meat thermometer. If the chicken looks done, then sticking the thermometer in and getting a reading of 75°C adds certainty to what you think you know.

If the chicken looks pink on the inside you're not going to eat it, no matter what the thermometer says. If it looks well done but the temperature is not reading high enough, you might be tempted to try measuring again in case the first reading was inaccurate. The thermometer doesn't directly tell you whether your food is safe. It simply provides added information to help you decide.

It is not simply a matter of developing more accurate tests. As tests become more sensitive, they also become more likely to falsely label something as a problem. Advancing technology starts to trade false negatives for false positives. Because they pick up and show every tiny thing, sometimes they can mislead us into thinking there is a problem when there isn't.

I once looked after a patient on the ward who had pneumonia that was worsening by the day. Someone suggested we do a CT scan to look for a blood clot in the lung vessels. When people are unwell and sitting around in hospital they can develop a blood clot that travels to the lungs.

We went ahead, and the scan reported a small clot in a small section of one lung. In our assessment it almost certainly was not the reason she was getting worse. But a clot had been found, and now we had to decide what to do about it. The normal treatment for blood clots is blood thinners, which carry the risk of causing bleeding. We know that the benefit of blood thinners outweighs the risk when the clot is big, but for small clots we don't have good data.

We started her on blood thinners. Two days later she had a cardiac arrest and we could not resuscitate her. Her post-mortem showed a bleed inside the brain, but no clot in her lungs.

It wasn't wrong to get the CT scan. It wasn't wrong for the radiologist to report a blood clot. It wasn't wrong for us to start her on blood thinners as a result. Tragically, the patient was simply a VOMIT: a Victim of Medical Imaging Technology.

Even if there had truly been a very small blood clot, we wouldn't have known what to do about it. Maybe we all walk around with tiny clots in our lungs from time to time that cause no harm? We don't go around scanning healthy people so there is really no way of knowing.

Currently various 'entrepreneurs' and media outlets are promoting the idea of screening healthy people for disease (mainly cancer) by doing full-body scans. What if the scan doesn't find any cancer, but it does find a small nodule in your body somewhere? This nodule is not causing you any harm, and most likely never will. But there is a tiny chance it might someday turn into cancer. Now that you know about it, do you take the risk of having a needle inserted into your body cavity in order to have it biopsied? Do you opt for an unnecessary operation to remove it because the doctor can't be sure what it is? Or do you watch and wait, living with the anxiety of knowing you have this unknown thing inside your body?

The only person who benefits here is the person making money from the scanner.

The public believe that more advanced testing equals better medical care. They expect expensive technology to get the diagnosis right 100 per cent of the time. It cannot.

Medicine in general cannot always get it right.

You might be horrified to learn that the medical profession expects to miss 1 per cent of cases with a life-threatening diagnosis. What if you're in the 1 per cent? But you don't see how much harm we would have to do to get that down any further. Cancers caused by radiation from scanners, or allergic reactions to contrast. We spend millions and millions of dollars every year following up patients with incidental findings from scans or blood tests and trying to figure out what to do with them. Many of these patients go on to have invasive procedures to work up the findings that end up harming them for no benefit.

We do our absolute best, and usually there is a good outcome, but other times nothing we can do is enough.

◆◆◆

I cannot leave a chapter about technology without mentioning the more mundane variety used for communications and administration. When I started as a house officer we were still operating with pagers and fax machines. Given that the public paging network was to be shut down in 2017, there was an impetus to move things along. Pagers are still alive and well in hospitals, but relegated to emergency functions rather than being standard issue. It was clear at the time that the network was in decline, as messages became increasingly garbled

— strings of unrelated letters and numbers. Sections of the message would get cut off.

One morning I received a page informing me that 'the patient in Bed 4 needs to be prescribed some anal##'.

I guessed it was meant to say 'analgesia'. I toyed with the idea of calling back and asking whether they wanted that on a regular or as-needed basis.

Fax machines took longer to be phased out. I surely cumulatively spent days of my life dealing with their capricious behaviour. You have an important referral to another specialty or a request for an urgent procedure to fax. You put it through the slanted tray at the top of the machine, only to be told you have to use the face-down scanner. If you had tried the scanner first, it would have been the tray you needed. You forget to press '5' first for an internal fax number, so it doesn't send.

You send it, but even though the screen says the fax was delivered, sometimes it just wasn't. Or it has been lost among the reams of paper that get thrown away because the messages don't get to the right person at the other end. Of course you don't know this until 4 p.m. because you've been attending to other patients, and you suddenly realise the people who were supposed to come see your patient haven't come. So much for 'Yeah, yeah, just fax us a referral.'

At least for inpatient services you did eventually realise. If you were sending a fax for some outpatient follow-up, you just prayed that the patient realised they hadn't had any communication from the hospital and called to enquire. You hoped nobody died because they were lost to follow-up due to an errant fax machine. In my heart I know this must surely have happened to somebody.

If you were sending an external fax, you might as well have folded your sheet of paper up into an aeroplane and thrown it out the window in the general direction.

While we have moved on from these relics, the more recent technology that we currently rely on also lets us down on a daily basis. The hospital's computer operating systems are all outdated. Some random character in the text of a discharge summary prevents it from being finalised and I spend an hour on the phone to IT trying to fix the problem. Then I press print and the printer jams, or the toner cartridge is low. This is time in my busy day I'll never get back.

The computer programs we rely on to be able to view patient documents, lab results and X-rays often crash. Every time I rotate to a different hospital there is something about my user account that has been set up incorrectly that takes days to resolve. You prescribe a long list of medications into the electronic medication chart, only for all your work to be lost in 'the loading screen of death' after you hit Prescribe.

Doctors sometimes find creative ways around these inconveniences to get the job done. I came across this entry in the notes of a patient I was seeing:

> Letter between I and P n keybard desnt wrk.
> Pain in abdmen was straight after cnstipatin.

Thankfully Health New Zealand Te Whatu Ora has prepared a robust response to the IT issues in hospitals. A week before Christmas 2024 they announced a proposal to cut 1120 full-time IT jobs around the country — almost half the IT workforce. They clearly felt they didn't need them anymore, following the recent rollout of a new patient tracking system in a major New Zealand hospital.

The system was designed to track where patients are in the hospital, which services and specialists they are admitted under, and log important patient details. Mostly it did, but not always. Friends told me that the $95 million project 'misplaced' patients, some of whom spent days in hospital before someone realised no doctors had come to see them. One day it listed all the babies on the postnatal ward as deceased. Junior doctor feedback was swift.

'This was the equivalent of a self-inflicted cyber-attack,' noted one.

'I have angry-cried four times during this rollout, which is more than I've cried in the last four years. I hate it so much. I hate this ghetto 40% off Briscoes sale deckchair excuse of a health system,' observed another.

These are not even the most obvious problems facing IT. New Zealand is supposed to have a nationwide integrated health system, yet if you travel to another region for medical care I can no longer access your records. Each city's hospitals have their own systems, which do not talk to each other, as we saw in Chapter 1.

7.

SOMETIMES BAD STUFF JUST HAPPENS

A doctor's confidence level is strongly tied to their recent successes or failures. I was working as the general medical registrar when the ED referral phone rang.

'Hi, it's Claire here from ED. Listen, I've got this 65-year-old man who has come in with left knee pain. I can't find any sinister explanation for it, and he's not unwell, but he can't safely mobilise so I can't send him home. I think he needs to be admitted for some pain relief and physiotherapy.'

'Sounds like an orthopaedic problem.'

'Yeah, ortho came and saw him; they said it's a quadriceps sprain. He's got pain and loss of strength on active hip flexion.'

'But they're not interested in looking after him?'

'Sadly not.'

'All right, that's fine. I'll go and say hi, and get the physio on to him.'

Burt was a cheery-looking man with a flabby double chin. He was sitting up reading the newspaper in his ordinary clothes. He slid his reading glasses down his nose to look at me as I walked into the room.

'Ah, you must be the doctor?'

'Guilty as charged! Nice to meet you, Burt.'

We shook hands.

'So what brings a healthy man like yourself to this hell-hole?'

He chuckled heartily.

'Well my left knee is playing up. I got out of bed this

morning and this pain just shot right down into my knee.'

'You just got out of bed like you would any other day? You weren't doing any stretching or exercising or anything else crazy?'

'No. No craziness in bed, not this week at least.'

He gave me a sly wink.

'We can come back to that later maybe,' I joked with him. 'Any other medical problems?'

'I take a blood thinner for my . . . I've got a heart arrhythmia.'

I nodded.

Inwardly I was starting to get that odd tingle, that chill in the spine, those slight goosebumps that told me I needed to be careful here. Something was not adding up. Usually people sprain their quads by excessive stretching or physical activity, not by getting out of bed in the morning.

'Right, let's have a look at this leg of yours. Might be easiest if you took your trousers off.'

I have always found it odd that people always comply with this request in an instant, even though they only met me five minutes earlier. Not in a weird way. Just in a way that reminds me how much trust is placed in us.

I stared at his knees, his thighs and his hips. All completely normal-looking. I was expecting to see at least a little puffiness on the left side, but both sides looked the same. I felt all around his knee, along his thigh and around his hip and could not feel any swelling. He was completely unbothered as I pressed deep into the tissues.

I pulled back the tissue on the outside of the knee and ran my hand along the inside edge of the kneecap, looking for a bulge to form back on the outside of the knee. Nothing. There was no fluid inside that knee joint.

I straightened my back and furrowed my brow.

'Okay, now straighten your leg and try to lift it up from the hip.'

'Argggh!'

He barely got his leg a few centimetres off the bed before it fell back down with a thud. Burt sat forward sharply, clutching his upper thigh in obvious agony.

The chill in my spine was getting stronger.

I picked up his observation chart. Stone-cold vital signs, nothing to suggest he was bleeding anywhere. His blood count was normal. And yet . . .

I told Burt I would be back shortly and went out to call the radiologist. I told him Burt's story.

'Sounds pretty unexciting. Probably a muscle sprain. Why do you want to do a CT scan?' The radiology registrar was clearly unimpressed.

'I'm worried about an iliopsoas bleed.'

'With a normal haemoglobin? And normal vital signs?' came the almost mocking reply.

'Yes.'

'I dunno, man, this is pretty weak.'

You haven't spent a day working in a public hospital unless you've had to cut through thickets of bush to get somewhere. Luckily, as you become more senior you acquire a bigger machete.

'All right,' I said. 'What's your name?'

'Why?'

'So I can document in the notes the name of the person who refused the scan.'

Silence as he pondered his options.

'All right, I'll put him through for a CT with contrast.'

The scan showed bleeding into his iliopsoas muscle. This beast of a muscle sits in your lower back and courses down through the pelvis to attach to the upper part of your thigh bone, where it helps to bend the hip.

I was pretty happy with myself. We usually didn't pick up iliopsoas bleeds until they became major and the patient was trying to die. We had got on to this early, so we could reverse his blood thinner and stop it from getting worse. He would have a good outcome.

I carried an internal swagger at work for the next couple of days. Master diagnostician, coming through!

◆◆◆

I was on my way to see a young man who had been sent to hospital by his GP with a vomiting bug. I had rolled my eyes when I got the phone call. Young healthy people don't need to be hospitalised for a vomiting bug. Take a concrete pill, try to keep down whatever fluids you can, and camp next to the toilet for the next 24 hours, like your grandparents would have done. I planned to give him a prescription for some anti-nausea tablets and oral rehydration solution, and send him home.

The young man was curled up in a ball on the bed.

'I just woke up this morning and I've been dry-retching all day!' he told me.

His head was hung over a vomit carton and every so often he would tense his shoulders and stick his neck out further, trying hard to expel something into the container but having no luck.

He was quite pale, and his upper lip was curled up into a sickly snarl.

'Have you vomited anything at all, or just retching?'

'Just retching.'

'Any diarrhoea?'

'No, no diarrhoea. Just a runny nose for the last few days.'

The thing that struck me was that he seemed very dehydrated. His heart rate was running along at 120, which is quite high for someone not exercising, and when I shook his hand to greet him I noticed his fingers were quite cold. These were both signs that not enough fluid was circulating in his blood. But if he hadn't vomited and had no diarrhoea, where would he have lost all that fluid?

I examined him from head to toe and couldn't find anything else abnormal.

The slight chill was starting to form in my spine again. I went and grabbed the ultrasound machine from the ED corridor next door. I turned on the probe marked Cardiac and the machine started clicking and whirring. I expected smoke to start billowing out the back at any second.

'I'm just going to have a look at your heart with this

ultrasound machine. It's like the one they use on pregnant women, but I'm hoping not to find that with you.'

Not even a chuckle. When patients don't laugh at my stupid jokes, I know they're truly unwell.

'Be warned, the ultrasound gel is really cold.'

He tensed up as I put the jelly-covered probe on his chest.

Up on the screen popped a black-and-white image of his beating heart. A normal heart looks small and vigorous, with the white outline of the edge of the heart muscle swinging back and forth across the screen as it pumps away. This guy's heart was big and feeble. Not much swinging. Just a tired-looking heart that was struggling to keep up and had slowed to a jog.

He sensed my disquiet and managed to crane his head up from the vomit carton to look at me.

'Found something?'

'I think you have inflammation of your heart muscle from a virus. It's called myocarditis.'

I paused to think about what I was going to say next.

'It's a very serious condition that can be fatal, so we need to act quickly. The good news is often we don't catch it early enough but we have with you, which gives us the best chance of getting on top of things.'

He swallowed hard. 'So is there some medication you can give me to fix it?'

'Not directly, but we can give you some medication to help your heart along. We'll also probably need to get you transferred to another hospital that specialises in this kind of thing so they can keep a close eye on you.'

He nodded seriously.

'Are your parents around?'

'They live an hour up north.'

'Is it okay if we call them to come down?'

'Yup. Yup, of course.'

There are two diseases that can hit an otherwise healthy young person in the morning and kill them by lunchtime: meningococcal disease and myocarditis. Both are rare, but they slink around under cover of darkness, two red eyes stalking you, impersonating other friendly creatures when you turn to look, and only pouncing when they are sure they have you.

I called my mate in intensive care and together we worked slickly over the next half-hour to insert a plastic catheter into the artery in the patient's wrist so we could monitor his blood pressure, and then a large, long catheter into the jugular vein in his neck so we could infuse powerful medications to stimulate his heart to beat harder, pumping more blood around his body.

We arranged for transfer to the local cardiovascular unit. Sometimes when the heart is severely affected people need to go on a heart bypass machine, which does the job of pumping the blood while the heart recovers. Those are only available at a few hospitals, not including this one. My friend and I were standing outside the room, waiting for the ambulance to arrive to pick him up. The young man was stable.

'Good job picking this up,' said my mate. 'It would

have been easy to dismiss as gastro, or flu, or just run-of-the-mill sepsis.'

I was quietly chuffed with myself.

'Well, you know, something just felt off.'

The overhead alarm went off. A stone dropped in my stomach.

We ran back into the room. Our patient was lying on the bed, pale and grey and gasping like a goldfish out of water.

I yanked an oxygen mask off the back of the bed, fumbled around with the tubing and rammed it onto the oxygen port. Then I cranked up the oxygen until there was a loud hissing coming from the wall. I slapped the mask onto the young man's face and started squeezing the inflatable bag attached to it to push air into his lungs. By now some ED nurses had rushed in and one of them knelt on the side of the bed and, fingers interlocked, started pushing down on the centre of the young man's chest with violent force. His blood pressure tracing, which had flatlined, began to register something with each push.

My mate stood at the foot of the bed, conducting the instrumentalists. His face had started to shine from sweat, but the voice that spread out over the orchestra pit was unflappable.

'Okay, our rhythm is VT.' (A ventricular tachycardia is an abnormally fast heartbeat.)

I looked up at the monitor. Instead of a nice organised electrical tracing with little spikes and pauses, there were large broad waves travelling across the screen, like a monster swell in the ocean, each one threatening to sink the little ship braving its waters.

'We need to deliver our first shock. Can we please charge the defibrillator.'

One of the nurses pressed the charge button. The machine issued a crescendoing whistle until it reached the required voltage, after which it held a steady whine.

'Okay, everybody stand back and let's deliver the shock.'

The sound that comes out when 200 joules is dumped into a patient is a dull thud. Their arms fling up into the air for a second like some kind of exorcism, although usually we're trying to keep the spirit inside the body rather than evict it.

'Okay, still in VT. Let's continue compressions.'

The person leading the resuscitation makes all the difference. If they panic, the whole room becomes a confused din of people talking and tripping over each other, with nobody knowing what's going on.

My mate was cool. On some occasions he has been known to pull up a chair and direct the efforts from his throne. The room was actually very quiet, given what was going on.

'Okay, Mary, I'd like you to take a blood gas for us. John, Savitha and Ellen, you three rotate on chest compressions. Princey, can you please start drawing up our adrenaline and amiodarone. Ivor, could you please intubate him.'

The nurses reported back calmly as they did their tasks. A couple of ED doctors came in to help as well.

We worked like this for 90 minutes. We threw everything we had at him. He had 40 shocks to try to restore his heart rhythm. He had the kitchen sink of anti-arrhythmia drugs. We carried on past the point of failure, because sometimes hope gets the better of us.

The waves kept rolling through. There was no pulse. Everyone in the room was drenched in sweat. Muscles were burning from doing compressions for an hour and a half. The floor was littered with plastic syringes and paper wrappings. Droplets of blood had flicked off and speckled the linoleum.

'Okay, everyone, I think further resuscitation is not going to be successful. Is anyone against stopping?'

Silent headshakes.

'Okay, stop CPR please.'

This moment is nothing like the way it is portrayed on TV. No one stands there and loudly declares the time of death. Everyone just starts silently packing up the rubbish, and slowly the room clears as everyone goes back to the other work that is waiting for them.

'Looks like the mum has just arrived. I'll go and talk to the family, eh?' my mate said to me. 'I'll catch up with you later.'

I wiped the sweat off my brow and nodded gratefully.

I walked down the corridor and back to the flight desk. Ten patients waiting to be seen. I picked up the nearest file. As I was walking into the room I heard muffled sounds coming from the resus corridor. The double doors opened briefly, probably as someone walked through, and her horrific primal howling echoed through the department. That kind of grief must rip every feeling out of your body. The sound pierced right into my soul.

I closed the curtain behind me.

'So, tell me about your diarrhoea.'

◆◆◆

At the end of my shift I passed through the ED waiting room, where the queue was almost out the door. I smiled politely at the people in line as I squeezed past them, shrugging my armpits tight so that they wouldn't be attacked by the sticky smell wafting from them.

I welcomed the cool breeze that hit my face as I stepped out into the night. Depending on the time of the year the breeze, or heat, or the smell of autumn leaves is nature's way of flushing out the burden of the shift from my brain and making room for normal life to fill it.

This time the events of the shift were slimy and congealed, difficult to wash away.

As I walked to the carpark I came across an empty Coke can on the pavement. I booted it as hard as I could. It made a loud ping and flew towards some nearby hydrangeas, ricocheted off the planter box, and rolled down some stairs.

I immediately felt guilty and went over to go pick it up. At the foot of the stairs and off to the side, hidden by more plants, my mate sat on a small bench. He was on call for a whole 24 hours and was out getting some fresh air.

I went and sat down.

'Fucking enterovirus, huh?' he said.

I grunted.

Enteroviruses are a common cause of myocarditis and the test had come back positive for our patient.

For a while we sat and listened to the low hum of cars exiting the carpark.

Finally I cleared my throat.

'What could we have done differently? Maybe I should have gone and seen him first, before my other patients. Then we could have got on to it sooner.'

My mate looked at me sideways.

'And I'm sure that if he had come in with a big sticker on his forehead that said "Myocarditis" you would have. But he didn't. And even if you had got on to it sooner, the only thing saving this guy was ECMO [the heart bypass machine]. There's no way we could have got him across [to the other hospital] in time before his heart stopped.'

I looked down at the ground.

'Yeah, but maybe . . .'

He started shaking his head.

'What's that rule in *The House of God*? The patient is the one with the disease?'

I nodded reluctantly.

'Sometimes bad stuff just happens.'

This is an important lesson for us all. Sometimes bad stuff just happens. You can make all the right decisions and still fail to avoid the bad shit. And your decisions can only be made with the information you have at the time.

◆◆◆

There is a perception among our profession that saying 'I don't know' is a weakness. That a doctor needs to exhibit certainty in order for patients to feel properly looked after.

I was a house officer on Dr Xavier's team. He was a wiry man with a grey moustache, and he always dressed in a suit, tie and vest to conduct his rounds, even when it was 30 degrees outside. The suit wanted to be noticed. The suit did not care about modern sensibilities, like infection control. When offered a gown to visit a patient with a multi-drug-resistant bacterium, Dr Xavier would simply extend his hand and give a firm shake of his head with his eyes closed. He'd go and drag his big floppy sleeves all over the patient while examining them, and then move on to the next patient, who was not (yet) covered in resistant bugs, and he would drag those same floppy sleeves over them.

Dr Xavier shuffled around the ward as he moved from patient to patient. We had patients on several floors of the hospital but Dr Xavier did not like to show any weakness and insisted on taking the stairs. We would have to pause at the end of each flight for a breather.

He joked that retirement meant having to listen to his wife nag him every day, which would lead to his death in less than a year. At least, we assumed it was a joke.

When the specialist does the ward round, the registrar or the house officer usually reprises the patient's details before you see them. Then the specialist sees the patient while the house officer writes detailed notes. The registrar is there to fill in any gaps and keep a note of all the important things that need to be done. Usually there are one or two medical students standing around as well.

One day the ward round dragged more than usual. While seeing the fifth patient, I was standing attentively with my pen hovering over the clinical notepaper, waiting for Dr Xavier to finish listening to the patient's lungs so he could tell me what he heard. My eyes wandered around the room. The patient wore Snoopy-themed socks. I snickered. The med students were preoccupied with their phones. The registrar was staring into space. An attractive nurse walked past and I stood up straighter and ran my hand through my hair.

Dr Xavier had been listening for quite a while. So attentively in fact that he had closed his eyes to better focus his hearing.

We all started to realise something was off when we noticed the patient had tucked his chin to his chest and was staring up and off to the side at Dr Xavier, who was slowly slumping down towards him.

The registrar cleared her throat sharply.

'Dr Xavier!'

He woke with a startle, shook his head rapidly from side to side and looked around sheepishly at all of us.

'... Right, and, yes, well, heart sounds are dual without murmurs, chest is clear throughout, as I was saying.'

He seemed pleased that he had done such a good job covering his tracks.

It was now 2 p.m. and we had three patients left to see. Dr Xavier delighted in quizzing the medical students along the way. He didn't seem to care that at the end of the ward round *he* might be finished, but *we* still had a lot more to do and daylight was rapidly running out.

I stared out the window as he started asking the students about Wilson's disease. The sunlight hit the roof of the carparking building opposite and splashed down over the road and courtyard below. It had soaked into the pavement and was trying to reach into the hospital to pull us into its warmth.

My foot almost left the ground as I fantasised about running towards the window and jumping through it, to gently float towards the ground while sparrows flitted around me. I picked out a random person I could see walking around below and scrunched my eyes closed, hoping some unknown superpower would switch my body with theirs.

'What do you think, Ivor?'

I was jolted from my daydream.

'Sorry, I'm sorry, I missed the question.'

'I said, if you think this is Wilson's disease, what test would you do to confirm that?'

'Umm, let me think. Ahh . . . copper level?'

Dr Xavier winced.

'No, no. You would do a serum ceruloplasmin.'

As we walked into the next patient's room he pulled me aside and whispered, 'Ivor, when you're answering a question, I don't care if you're right or wrong, but for the love of god, sound confident. Patients don't like an unsure doctor.' He winked at me.

◆◆◆

The problem with certainty is that we work in an inherently uncertain field, so sooner or later you will be wrong, and then the patient will lose trust. As you make your way through med school and specialty training, educated guesswork is encouraged.

As part of training in intensive care, you rotate through other specialties that provide relevant experience. It is kind of like being on loan from one sports club to another. One of these specialties is anaesthesia. While I was a senior trainee in my own specialty, for a few months I was a 'baby' anaesthesia trainee. (They are known as baby anaesthesia trainees not because they work with babies, but because they are just starting out.) They work with a different specialist every day, and because they are newbies and eager to make a good impression, they have to tolerate that specialist's particular idiosyncrasies. If the specialist tells them they must always place the drug label longways on the syringe, they would affirm this notion by indicating that only a cretin would think to place it any other way. The next day, when a different specialist tells them the label must always go horizontally, they would say exactly the opposite. Shit sandwiches must be eaten with a smile.

I was in quite a different position. When it came to

impressing people, I had crossed the *x*-axis on the 'giving a shit' graph. I just had to serve out the term of my loan and not do anything egregious along the way.

One day I was with a particularly curmudgeonly anaesthetist. He was also, unfortunately, very good at his job. I had arrived 15 minutes early to draw up all the drugs for our first case. The patient was still in pre-op. The specialist limped into the operating theatre with a dour look on his face, threw his bag on the nearest chair, and made his way towards me.

I summoned up some enthusiasm from somewhere in my heels.

'Good morning, my name's Ivor. I'm working with you today!'

He nodded his head upwards, then regarded my drug tray.

'That's not the way I draw them up.'

He discarded the contents of my drug tray and started drawing them up from scratch.

This is going to be a long fucking day, I thought.

'Haven't seen you before, Ivan, how far along in your training are you?'

I winced.

'I'm the ICU trainee. I'm spending a year with the department.'

'ICU, huh? You're a fan of self-abuse, are you?'

I said nothing.

Later, after we had got the patient off to sleep, we were sitting in front of the monitor. He was explaining how to give the perfect anaesthetic. He got on to the topic of some rarely used drug I cannot now recall the name of. Let's call it obscurium.

'So, what is the half-life of obscurium?' he asked me.

I placed both palms on my chin and rubbed my eyes with my fingertips.

'Not sure.'

He frowned.

'You're not going to venture a guess?'

'Look, I really don't know.'

'Most trainees would at least say something. Just think of it from first principles.'

'What is the point of me making a random guess when I have no idea?'

A vein on his forehead was starting to bulge.

'To show you're engaged.'

'I *am* engaged. I just don't think there's any point throwing out some number for no good reason.'

'So you won't answer my question.'

'I guess not.' I stared at him defiantly.

'Well, I won't give you the answer then. I'm not here to spoon-feed you.'

'Okay.'

We spent the rest of the morning in silence.

◆◆◆

The medical profession has come a long way in terms of being prepared to admit fallibility.

When laparoscopic gallbladder surgery first arrived in New Zealand in the 1990s, a well-respected surgeon accidentally injured the patient's spleen during one of the early cases and the spleen had to be removed. When the surgeon saw the patient the next morning he explained that the operation had been successful. As he was walking out of the room he stopped at the door, turned around and said, 'Oh, and we had to take out your spleen too,' before rushing away.

His registrar was left to pick up the pieces.

These days doctors are more willing to admit that they are human, but there is still a lot of taboo around displaying uncertainty to the public. And yet I firmly believe patients want honesty.

This is one of the mistakes I believe New Zealand made with the messaging around vaccination during the Covid pandemic. Any medical treatment involves benefit and risk, and the benefits of the vaccine far outweighed the risks, but we were so determined to reap the former that we downplayed the latter to the public.

We infantilised the public, thinking people wouldn't cope with an honest discussion. So we talked only about the good stuff. Then, when a few people started experiencing some of the downsides we hadn't told them about, the public started losing trust.

This is why snake-oil salesmen and alternative health practitioners are so popular. Their products don't work for much other than muscular aches and pains, so on a biological level they can't have any downsides. They can make outrageously confident claims without losing people's trust.

Conventional medicine has biological effects, and these go hand in hand with side-effects. It is like sunshine and rain: you can't have one without the other. Conventional medicine cannot get away with false certainty. If you offer certainty in an uncertain situation, you set yourself up to fail.

To judge a decision by its outcome is a mortal sin of logic, but people often do. Armchair experts judge every decision that was made during an unprecedented pandemic through the lens of knowing the future. With hindsight, they conclude that decisions must have been bad because bad outcomes occurred. The economy suffered, so therefore a bad decision must have been made.

They lose sight of the fact that during the pandemic, maintaining 'normality' was not an option. Big decisions had to be made, which risked delivering good outcomes or bad outcomes, and no one knew at the time which it would be.

You work with all the information you can gather, and make a call. And there will always be plenty who sit in their armchairs and mouth off if you get it wrong. They're not the ones who make any decisions of importance, but they have plenty of advice for those who do.

8.

ARSEHOLES, INCOMPETENTS & A FRAUDSTER

My friend Ken and I were starting on our surgery rotation as final-year medical students at a hospital we'll call Willowsea. Each surgical team of registrars, house officers and medical students works under several specialists, and one of them was a man of great importance. Let's call him Professor Plum.

We were scheduled to go into theatre that afternoon to watch one of his surgeries. We were both a bit nervous — not because we were eager to make a great first impression, but because of the stories we had heard about this man.

We turned up to theatre at 1 p.m. and were unceremoniously ushered into a corner of the room by one of the scrub nurses.

'The med students are here!' she proclaimed.

The professor was seated at the head of a patient covered in sterile drapes. His thick eyebrows slanted down towards a point above his large crooked nose, making him look like a hawk, and his lips were so thin they were almost invisible. A patchy grey beard completed the framing of his sneering visage.

He did not acknowledge us. Ken and I looked at each other uncertainly. We were too far away to see anything, but dared not move any closer without invitation. We were living, breathing totem poles.

Eventually the professor muttered to us in a gruff voice, without looking up from his work, 'Well, come closer then.'

We shuffled forward.

'You,' he said, pointing my way. 'What's your name?'

'Ivor.'

'Ivor?'

'Yeah.'

'Where's that from then?'

I swallowed hard, as I knew where this was going. Just be self-deprecating and don't take anything to heart, I told myself.

'I was born in Croatia.'

'Ah, you're a Yugoslav then? When did you come here?'

'1994.'

He rocked back and forth slightly, nodding as he pondered.

'You would have left in a hurry then, I imagine. Did they chase you out with a gun or a knife?'

A few people around the room chuckled.

I laughed along as if I was in on the joke.

'Ha, not sure.'

'Probably both. Once those cheap Russian AK-47s jammed, they probably had to resort to throwing knives.'

Oh, hilarious. I laughed out loud in an attempt to show I wasn't bothered, but I felt as if the entire room could see through my act. I felt my face burning up.

What he had said was not that bad. My friends said worse to me all the time. But they had that privilege because they had known me for so long. This eagle-faced fuck was not my friend. He had just met me and he was insulting me, trivialising my story in a room full of strangers. And actually, he knew nothing. They didn't use Russian AKs in the Yugoslav wars.

It turned out I was just the entrée, however.

'How about you?' he motioned to Ken.

'I'm Ken.'

'Ken? Well, that's going to be too hard to remember. I can never remember all the Chinese students' names. I'll call you Bill.'

Ken opened and closed his mouth a few times and stared blankly back.

We had both heard that this was the professor's modus operandi. He assigned any Asian student the names Bill or Bob. But we'd never seen it first-hand so we'd hoped it was just urban legend.

The professor spent longer with Ken. He asked about which school he went to and what his parents did. He was trying to establish whether Ken's family were 'rich Asians' or not. Ken's parents were immigrants who owned a takeaway shop.

As the conversation went on, Ken drifted closer and closer to the professor so that he could hear what the man was saying through his mask. Eventually, the professor side-eyed him and said, 'Get any closer and I'll send you right back to the takeaway store!'

Ken stared down at his feet. I will never forget the hurt I saw in his eyes.

I was enraged. I wanted to reach across and slap the professor's face, but I stood paralysed. I looked around the room, trying to catch the eye of someone else who was similarly incensed, but they all seemed to be going about their business, or even joining in and laughing. Then I locked eyes with one of the scrub nurses, who shook her head and whispered, 'Don't worry. It's just him.'

But actually it wasn't just him. It was all the enablers around him who turned a blind eye and normalised his actions. The standard you walk past is the standard you accept.

◆◆◆

The enablers are like the guards of a concentration camp. They don't conceive or carry out the terrible behaviour, but without them it could not be accomplished.

Some would argue that this is just hazing — a way of welcoming newcomers to the club. A little shit-talk among friends. It's an opportunity to show your mental toughness. After all, if a little verbal abuse unseats you, how will you handle the stress of plugging a bleeding vessel at three in the morning?

This kind of false equivalence is used to justify all manner of abuse against trainees and ensure their silence — not just in the medical realm. You're not my friend and I didn't sign up to the military, I would think.

Having a thick skin is important in our job, but should anyone have to put up with abuse? Sometimes it's a fine line.

◆◆◆

Many years ago I was called down to the ED to assist with a patient who needed to be admitted to the ICU. The middle-aged woman had been found unconscious at home that morning.

The ambulance officers wheeled her in to the resus bay. Her head was rolled over to one side and drool was coming out of the corner of her mouth.

'Suspected meningococcal disease,' they said in their handover.

The ED doctor and I looked at each other, then back at the patient. Sure enough, she was covered in purply-red splotches on her arms, legs and body.

I had a sudden vision of the ad campaigns that used to run when I was child, at the time of the meningococcal epidemic, telling Mum and Dad to press down on the rash with a glass, and if it didn't go away you needed to get your child to hospital. No matter how much experience or knowledge I had gained in medicine since, my instinct was still to look around for a glass.

The rash is a sign that the blood is starting to lose the ability to clot, and so there is bleeding under the skin surface.

Meningococcus is a bacterium that invades the lining of the brain causing meningitis, but also enters the bloodstream causing septicaemia. The major organs start to shut down and the blood stops clotting properly. Fluid seeps out of the blood vessels and fills the lungs. It is so fast that you can be healthy at breakfast, have the sniffles by lunch, and be dead by afternoon tea.

I pressed down hard with my knuckles on the centre of the patient's chest to see whether she could sense pain and respond normally. This manoeuvre looks brutal but can tell us a lot. Every time I go to do it I always hesitate slightly, remembering that a mate ended up being slated for it by a patient's family member in the *Woman's Weekly*.

The woman barely flinched.

In the ICU we prepared to put a breathing tube down her windpipe.

Intubating patients is something you need to do several hundred times before you are decent at it. Most of the time it is straightforward. You use a curved metal blade to lift the tissues at the back of the mouth, which lets the vocal cords pop into view. The plastic tube then slides in along the back of the mouth and into the cords.

But sometimes it's not straightforward. You need to administer powerful sedatives in order to carry out the procedure, and these make the patient stop breathing. Now they are relying on you to supply oxygen. Without oxygen, the brain can survive only about five minutes.

I was a newbie at the time, so Dr Mac came to help me.

Dr Mac was notoriously difficult to pin down. Rumour was that he had worked at the hospital so long he knew all the back corridors, and used them to his advantage. He would pop up suddenly behind your back like a poltergeist. However, his skill was undisputed: there was no human orifice into which it was too difficult for this man to insert a tube.

I had gathered all my equipment and was running through a checklist as I stood at the head of the bed with an oxygen mask held to the patient's face.

'All right, you ready?' asked Dr Mac.

'No, just give me a . . .'

But he had already started pushing drugs into the patient's IV line.

'Okay, drugs are in.'

'Umm, okay, ah . . .'

'Well, go on, have a look then.'

'But it hasn't been 45 seconds.'

'She's already fasciculating [involuntary muscle twitching]. Look! Go on, stick the blade in.' He motioned at me with his eyebrows.

I put the blade in her mouth and lifted it up to try to get the vocal cords in view.

Dr Mac had come around to stand beside me.

'Well? What do you see?'

'To be honest, I'm struggling to get a good view here, Dr Mac.'

'Well, fuck off then!'

A colossal force sent me careening off to the side, arms and legs flailing like the wacky inflatable man in front of the vacuum store. Dr Mac had hip-checked me, with the full momentum of his body catching me like a wrecking ball. He had managed to snatch the blade out of my hand in the same motion.

Recovering my balance (recovering my dignity would take longer), I looked over to see him digging around in the patient's mouth, cursing gruffly under his breath.

I looked up at the beeping monitor. Blood pressure 60/20. Oxygen level 85 per cent. Not good.

Then, 'I'm in,' he proclaimed, to my relief.

We started pushing oxygen through the tube and slowly the numbers on the monitor improved.

I looked at Dr Mac and asked sheepishly, 'So what kind of view did you get?'

'It was shithouse, but I just aimed in the direction I knew it should go.'

'Oh. Okay.'

I knew he was not trying to humiliate me. He was responding to an urgent situation. My thick skin was developing apace.

◆◆◆

Can a doctor who is a dick to colleagues still be a good doctor? I would argue not, because nobody works in a silo in a hospital setting. If a big-shot wants his plans to be executed he has to rely on his 'minions'. And if the minions are scared of being humiliated — well, that doesn't lead to good communication among the team, which inevitably compromises care.

Doctors get away with bullying and humiliation and outright abuse of junior staff because of the silence of their colleagues. Silence leads to female trainees crying in the locker room after work because a surgeon got in real close in theatre and started pushing up against their breasts. Or because they are being pushed for sex in exchange for career advancement, and know that making a big deal out of it will stop their career dead in its tracks.

Senior doctors get up to all kinds of seedy things: sexual harassment; sex with medical students on the promise of good grades; providing a good character reference in court for a trainee who committed a crime because 'he's a good trainee and a conviction would damage his career'; doing cocaine with their colleagues at weekends.

If you've been around the yard enough times, you know exactly who has a reputation for what. Ironically, many abusers are well liked and respected as scholars and educators.

My own specialty, intensive care, is not immune from accusations of toxic workplace culture and bad behaviour. It's everywhere. A lot of problems have been reported in the news over the years, and some intensive care units have lost their privileges to train junior doctors for a period of time because of it.

It's only a handful of individuals doing the offending. But, as the saying goes, a few bad apples can ruin the whole barrel. And some individuals who have encrusted themselves within the system over the years can be hard to get rid of.

Firstly, there's quite a high barrier separating the things everybody knows happen from the things that are legally provable. Attempts to fire doctors in the past have backfired because they have hired good lawyers, and actual evidence is hard to obtain. Victims often don't want to talk publicly.

Say you know your colleague is a sordid character — perhaps you know from experience — but they are one of your partners in private practice, and together you bring in good money. Are you going to risk your own welfare and future by trying to bring them down, or are you going to ignore what doesn't directly affect you?

Most importantly, and most directly related to the point of this book, the health system is a beggar on the streets, holding a hand out for scraps. With shortages of specialists in every field, the public system is indebted to anybody that helps to keep it going, especially those who bring in extra funding or who are well-known figures, so their shine polishes anything close to them. Going after them for 'character flaws' would be like a one-legged person shooting themselves in the remaining foot.

The system is not ignorant; it just chooses to ignore.

Everyone knows the feeling of being in a stressful situation. Maybe you're anxious because you have to give a public speech. Maybe you're in a situation where you're fearing for your life. Your vision starts to blur at the edges. Someone near you says something and you don't hear them. Your entire focus is on the 'threat' in front of you, and your mind clears away any other thoughts.

That is the state of the health system right now. It has no capacity to deal with anything other than limping along and trying to survive. Any fodder that fills a gap is good enough.

This means bad actors are even less likely to be brought to heel.

I worked once with a general medical specialist who was not an arsehole but was a terrifyingly bad doctor. He sported black spiky hair and a baseline vacant facial expression. He spoke quickly and in a way that sounded as if he was swallowing half of his words, so everyone had to lean in to hear him. When he got excited about something — and this was often as he led himself into dark alleyways devoid of logic when discussing patient management — he spoke twice as fast.

He was so bad, one registrar had resigned on finding out they were allocated to this man's team for three months.

And yet it was impossible to feel real hostility for the guy because he was the nicest person on earth. His quiet tone and his malproportioned eyes reminded you of a sad puppy.

He had been employed in the midst of increasing vacancies in the general medical department, and it didn't take him long to make a name for himself.

It was on the back of many horror stories, which sadly I can't tell here, that I dragged my feet to this specialist's ward on a Monday morning, with three days of relieving for his sick registrar to look forward to. I wondered whether she was actually ill or had just taken a mental health break.

The specialist had clinic that morning so he told us to see the patients, then meet with him later in the morning to discuss them. We all sat down at 11 a.m., printed patient lists in hand, and I braced myself for the hurricane that was about to hit.

'So, Mrs Gould,' I began. 'The neurologist saw her this morning and thinks the weakness in her legs doesn't fit any pattern and is probably related to stress from her recent traumatic childbirth. Anyway, she's recovered and we saw her walking around the ward this morning. I think she can go home.'

'Okay, yes, discharge today,' said the specialist. 'But we should order an outpatient MRI of the spine.'

'Umm, okay. Why?'

'Well, it might be an epidural haematoma [bleeding around the spinal cord] from the epidural.'

'I don't think she'd improve spontaneously if that was the case.'

'We should just make sure.'

'Okay. So if you're worried about blood around her spinal sac, shouldn't we be keeping her in hospital and doing it urgently?'

'No, no. I think she can go home if neurology is happy.'

'Okay . . . Right. Well, Mrs Fen next door is doing better with physio in the last 24 hours, but she's on a bit of oxygen today and feels more breathless. Examination shows she's fluid overloaded, so I've given her a touch of diuretic.'

He nodded at me seriously. 'You know, we really have to consider fat embolism here.'

'Fat embolism?'

'Yes, she's had a fracture of the ASIS, so that could lead to fat embolism.'

The ASIS is the pointy part of your hips that you can feel when you press off to the side and below your belly button, just above your hip joint. It is commonly fractured in old people during a fall, but it is only a tiny fragment of bone that breaks. Fat embolism happens when you break a major bone like your leg or thigh, and the fat from the bone marrow seeps into your bloodstream and travels to your lungs. It has to be a big bone, with a lot of marrow in it.

'I'm not sure that's a big enough bone to cause fat embolism . . .'

'Okay, well, it's just something to consider.'

'Okay.'

'She's also high risk for a PE [a blood clot in the lung]. Let's treat her for that.'

I coughed to hide the growl of derision that was making its way out.

'You mean put her on high-dose blood thinner?'

'Yes. It's highly likely she has a PE.'

'Do you want to do a scan to confirm that diagnosis?'

'No, I think just treat her.'

'Right.'

We then went on to talk about Mr Adams, who'd had a fall.

'We should ask surgery to come and stitch up the skin tear on his leg,' offered the specialist.

'It's a very superficial tear in fragile skin. I don't think suturing it is really going to be possible.' Which was a polite way of saying, 'Are you fucking crazy?'

'We should still get them to come have a look.'

'Okay.'

'And we should ask endocrinology for advice about his thyroid medication.'

I breathed in sharply. I wasn't sure if I could maintain the façade of politeness any longer.

'But aren't you an endocrinologist? Isn't that your second specialty?'

After he left, I took my house officers to a different room, out of earshot of anybody.

'Send Mrs Gould home; no MRI. Don't start Mrs Fen on blood thinners but send her down for a scan. Don't bother talking to surgery about Mr Adams, but call endo. Maybe don't mention the name of our consultant. Or actually, you know what? Do mention it. I actually don't care.'

They nodded. They had been on the team for a couple of months already; they knew the drill.

That afternoon I sent an email to some higher powers asking to meet.

We sat down in their cramped office the next day and I told them all these stories, and more.

'All this happened in just 24 hours. I don't think this person is competent to be employed as a specialist.'

They took my concerns down in writing, but it was to no avail.

◆◆◆

Other similarly useless doctors exist, and we have the legal profession to thank in part for the fact that some are still practising. If you have a good lawyer it is very hard to get fired for incompetence. The threshold of proof of patient endangerment is high, and unfair workplace practices and workplace discrimination are frequently cited by lawyers as reasons for poor performance. The Medical Council itself only seems to act in the most egregious offences, usually bordering on criminality.

Of course there needs to be protection against frivolous complaints, and to stop your job being on the line because a medical event ends badly. But the tree has grown so large that its branches now provide shade to the incompetent and abusive.

I put myself at risk, as have many registrars before and after me, in going against the advice of a specialist. But I put myself at risk in order to protect patients. We should not have to do that in a world-class health system.

◆◆◆

On the upside, at least these people are actually qualified...

When I was in medical school we were called to an urgent end-of-day class meeting towards the end of our third year. We were told there had been an imposter in our midst for the last three years. Jaran (not his real name) had been turned down for medical school. Rather than moving on and finding another career, or trying again in a couple of years, he turned up to campus and attended class with the rest of us who had been accepted. He threw himself fully into campus life. He was part of the student social committee, he was well liked by his classmates, and he even had a girlfriend in the same intake.

He would turn up to exams and mill around in the waiting room beforehand with the rest of us. Just before it was time to go in, he would excuse himself to pop to the toilet. Then he would slip out in the commotion as everybody surged through the open doors into the exam room. We only figured this out after the fact, when we compared notes. People remembered occasions when they were late to exams and, while making a mad dash from the carpark, they saw Jaran heading in the wrong direction.

Towards the end of our third year we started going into hospitals once a week to get hands-on experience with real patients. This was the transition period between the first half of the degree, which is completely theoretical, and the fully practical second half. We each received a shiny pin-on badge that we wore proudly over the left breast: 'Name Name, Student Doctor'.

Jaran called the badge manufacturer directly and complained that they had mistakenly not sent him his one. They apologised and posted it in the mail.

He was found out when his friends submitted a group lab assignment, listing him as one of the contributors. I can just imagine some poor postgraduate student, scrounging some extra cash by agreeing to mark medical school microbiology lab assignments, sitting there hunched over a desk late at night, weary face illuminated by a solitary lamp in an otherwise dark room, thinking, 'Who the hell is this Jaran guy?' Little did they know they were about to unmask a fraudster.

Class members took the news in many different ways. Those of us who didn't know him very well cracked jokes. Those who had been his close friends, and more, struggled with the deep betrayal. At least one person decided to benefit by selling the story to the *New Zealand Herald*. (It wasn't me.)

All of us contemplated the reasons for his years-long ruse. Was he just terrified of telling his parents he had failed, and a small lie eventually ballooned out of control? Or was he one of those pathological liars who deceive others as a way of life?

Whatever the circumstances, the medical school decided not to press any charges. Soon after, Jaran left a cryptic message on social media, not admitting to any wrongdoing. He said he had been offered a place in medical school in Australia, and would see us in the future.

After a while he faded from memory for most of us.

Ten years later my wife and I were having dinner with friends. Mosham was a GP with whom I had gone to medical school and we had been in the trenches together as first-year house officers. His wife was a nurse, and I had worked with her during one of my many rotations.

We were enjoying rich pasta at a charming brick-clad Italian restaurant in Ponsonby.

Mosham stopped halfway through a bite.

'Oh, something really weird happened the other day.'

'Yeah?' I said, head bent over and focusing on slurping my pasta without getting sauce on my shirt.

He didn't say anything. My wife elbowed me in the side and I looked up and saw Mosham was waiting for me to pay attention.

'Sorry, you were saying?'

'I've got this patient who I referred to a respiratory clinic a while back for treatment of bronchiectasis. She was seen last week, and today I get a clinic letter from the registrar who saw her.'

'Okay,' I said, taking another mouthful.

He pulled out his phone. 'Look at the name of the person who signed the letter.'

He showed us a screenshot.

> ... I have arranged for a follow up appointment in six months.
>
> Yours sincerely
>
> Jaran Jaranson
>
> Respiratory Research Fellow

I felt the hairs on my arms prickle.

'No . . . Surely not?!'

'It's weird, right?'

'His name's not that uncommon. There could be a bunch of docs out there with the same name.'

Mosham had started shaking his head before I had even finished my sentence, and had a triumphant smile on his face.

'Yeah, except there aren't. I searched the name on the Medical Council register. There's nobody by that name.'

My fork dropped on my plate with a loud clang.

He continued. 'I searched up the Australian register too. Same thing.'

'Wow.'

We held a long silence as our wives looked at each other, shrugging their shoulders. We explained the backstory.

'There's got to be a simple explanation,' I said. 'Maybe it's someone who is registered under their birth name, but uses a different name professionally.'

'Yeah, possibly.' Mosham seemed unconvinced.

'I mean, if it is him, why would he come back to the place where everybody knows him, and knows he's a fraudster, without at least changing his name? Surely no one is that stupid?'

'Maybe he actually went and graduated med overseas, and now he's come back to prove everyone wrong? And he registered under a different name, like you say, so that they wouldn't be able to find any reference to what happened at med school if they googled him.'

'But he wouldn't have had time to get through training and be a fellow already, would he?'

'These research positions are often labelled as fellow, but actually it's registrars who get employed in them, so the timing could fit.'

We slowly nodded at each other.

The food was getting cold.

'Anyway,' Mosham concluded, 'I emailed the Medical Council telling them about it. We'll see what they have to say.'

I lay awake until 3 a.m. doing investigative work on my phone. I figured there was probably some innocuous explanation and we were letting our imaginations run wild. The chances of this guy pulling the same stunt, with the same name, in the same city must be minuscule. Maybe, though, that's exactly the reason someone might try to pull it off.

A weird excitement built up in my stomach, a sense of intrigue that kept me googling even as my eyelids grew so viscous they barely let in any of the blue light from my phone. I felt like a detective following a trail.

My working theory was that he had graduated in medicine overseas under an assumed identity, and registered with the Medical Council back in New Zealand under that name, while using his real name in his day-to-day work. I deduced that soon after leaving New Zealand he had been accepted to a university in Australia, although I wasn't sure for what degree. I couldn't find his name in any med school graduation lists. He then surfaced some years later at a medical school in Poland, but again there was no record of him having graduated. He seemed to be using his real name at this time. Then the trail went dark.

About a month later Mosham texted me.

'Look at the news,' he said.

I opened the *Herald* home page. I was so agitated that the words on the screen blurred together, but I could still make out 'fake doctor' in the headline.

Reality turned out to be more far-fetched than our imaginings.

It was indeed him. He had flunked out of school in Poland and returned to New Zealand where he worked as a Covid contact tracer. At this job he told everybody he had trained as a doctor at Boston University and was waiting for his Medical Council application to go through. He even gave a presentation, detailing his experiences of working through the pandemic in Boston.

Around this time he appeared in court on a reckless driving charge, but was discharged after successfully arguing that a conviction would affect his career prospects. He produced bogus letters of support from the Medical Council and others.

He then got the job as a respiratory research fellow using a forged Medical Council practising certificate. He had been seeing patients in this job for six months before one of his letters made its way to my friend's inbox.

9.

BLOOD, SWEAT & TEARS

'How can there not be enough checks and balances to prevent fake doctors practising in New Zealand?' was the public outcry after the Jaran story hit the news.

Junior doctors are recruited by regional employment agencies or 'RMO units', which also handle rostering, leave requests and many other aspects of a junior doctor's working life. (The term junior doctor applies to any doctor who is not yet a qualified specialist. Some 'junior' doctors have been practising medicine for over 15 years.)

The recruiters have the unenviable job of trying to plug gaps in a wooden hull that is being ravaged by rot. The only surprising thing about forged documents making it through the vetting process is that it hasn't happened more often. It's a thankless task and recruiters last about as long as a bad smell on a windy day.

When I was a house officer I had a colleague called Alan.

Alan was a down-to-earth guy. He got up every morning at five to go for a run, yet always came into work perfectly groomed. His hair was held up and off to the side with wax and I had never seen a single strand out of place, even on a windy day. His shirts always had striking patterns, nice cuffs and were perfectly ironed.

Patients and nurses adored Alan's style, and he was so pleasant to everyone he made the rest of us look like jerks. Not that you could ever hold that against him. I had never seen Alan show frustration or annoyance. He remembered names upon hearing them once, and would enquire after your grandma who you had mentioned in passing two months previously. I often mused that Alan had so much goodness in him, it must seep out through his skin and keep him clean without ever needing to shower.

One day I was sitting outside the RMO unit in our hospital, waiting to discuss some aspect of my roster. I heard voices from within getting louder. Soon I realised it was Alan in there talking to one of the recruiters.

'Yes, I realise you don't usually approve leave requests at such short notice, but like I said, my father passed away this week. It's his funeral.'

'Okay, but we don't have anyone available to cover your shift this weekend.'

'So you're saying I *have* to come in and work it?'

'If you can find someone to cover your shift then we can grant your leave.'

'You're joking?'

'No, the service is very understaffed at the moment and short of relievers.'

There was a third-trimester pause before Alan continued, and I imagined him speaking through tightened lips. 'I don't know how many ways to say this. My dad just died. I won't be coming in to work this weekend. Goodbye.'

The door flew open. I opened my mouth to offer my condolences about his father but he flew past, his face bright red and an errant hair on his head sticking off to the side.

I have known RMO units to not infrequently breach

employment law. Declining leave requests without citing a reason, declining days in lieu (which must be granted as long as sufficient notice is given), asking doctors to find cover for their own leave, and rostering them in excess of the permitted hours. Then they take months to process overtime claims; that is if they get to them at all.

They are trying to keep the ship afloat by telling the slaves to row harder, except the underdeck is already half flooded. They rely on doctors not knowing their rights, or being too timid to insist on them. No wonder no one lasts long in the recruiter's job. It doesn't take long for the pressure from above and the kickback from below to squeeze them out. You just get used to emailing one recruiter, then after a few months you get the following automated reply: 'This person no longer works for the organisation.'

A rookie enters the picture, filled with bravado and the self-confidence that they will be able to keep these troublesome junior doctors in line. But their tyres were never designed for this kind of gravel. Soon they'll be off the road too.

The recruiters are simply following the directive of the hospital service managers. The managers themselves have little control over the understaffing and underfunding, but shit rolls downhill, as they say. To them we are disposable cogs in the machine.

They send emails telling us we need to stagger our dinner breaks in case there is an emergency. Never mind the fact that we all carry emergency pagers. Never mind the fact that there is hardly ever a doctor sitting around on every single ward in the hospital in case something happens.

We get texts like this from our managers:

> Hospital at capacity today, remember to ask yourself whether your patients are ready for discharge, and prioritise seeing all dischargeable patients first.

I am tempted to text back to ask whether they have reminded the police to make sure to catch the bad guys, or asked teachers to please prioritise the children.

When I was a house officer we had pagers, and if your pager went off on a busy ward round, even if you were with a sick or complex patient, you had to peel away from the team and find a landline. You hit the jackpot if you received both a succinct message and an extension to call back on. Usually, it was just an extension number. You had no idea of the seriousness of the issue until you called them. They might want a prescription for laxatives, or to tell you your patient had died. That's if you actually managed to reach the nurse who had paged you, which was not guaranteed.

On one occasion my pager went off and I scoured the central hub. No free landlines. I snuck into the orthopaedic plastering room, where I knew there was a phone tucked away in a corner behind some plaster of Paris mixing tins.

I dialled the extension I'd been given.

The phone rang and rang.

I gave up and went to rejoin the team. Sticking my head through the patient's curtain, I saw him sitting up eating a sandwich, with headphones on. There was nobody else in the room. He looked up at me with a pleasant sort of confusion.

'Would you like some?'

He offered me a triangle of bread, tomatoes and ham from the brown bag on the bed.

'No, I'm all right, thanks. I'm looking for the doctors who were here a minute ago.'

'Oh.' He looked disappointed. 'They went off that way.'

'Right, thanks. See you later, sir.'

'Cheerio then.'

I strode down the corridor. They couldn't have got far. My pager shrieked again. I picked it up and saw the same extension.

'Be nice if you told me what you fucking wanted!' I shouted at the machine.

I jogged back to the plaster room and dialled the number.

'Hello?' someone answered.

'Hi, this is Ivor, with Team B, returning a page.'

'Who are you after?'

'I don't know. They paged me.'

'Oh, right. Let me see if I can find who it was.'

I stared at the wall while waiting, listening to a lot of muffled shouting on the other end. Finally the line started to crackle again.

'Hello, this is Mary, charge nurse.'

'This is Ivor from Team B. You paged me?'

'Yes. Now, where are you? Mr Anderson is waiting to be discharged.'

'We haven't finished the round yet. We're still downstairs.'

'I paged you half an hour ago!'

'What time was that?'

'11.30!'

I checked my pager.

'Yes, you sent a page that said "Patient ready to be discharged, awaiting papers". I had no idea who that was about and you didn't leave a number.'

She muttered something unintelligible. 'Well, fine, but you wrote that he was for discharge this morning, so you should know about it.'

'Yes, but we have other patients to see first. I'll do the papers as soon as the round is finished.'

'Can't you just split off for a second and do them now?'

'No.'

'Okay, well, please hurry. The family are here and getting impatient.'

'Look, why doesn't he just go and we can mail him his papers?'

'He needs a new prescription.'

'Well, he'll just have to wait for now unfortunately.'

'You realise the hospital is full today, right? Discharges need to be prioritised.'

'Thanks for reminding me.'

I jogged back down the corridor and spent another good five minutes searching behind bed curtains to find my team again.

We finished the round at 12.30 and, dehydrated from a whole morning of walking and talking, I stopped to grab a quick drink. Then I headed upstairs to attend to Mr Anderson's discharge summary.

As I walked into the ward, cup in hand, Mary was standing at the receptionist's desk. When she saw me she puffed up her chest and raised her hand in the air as if she was about to discipline me physically.

'Off having a cuppa while the patients are waiting to go home, are we?'

I fantasised about giving her an earful, but just in time I recalled one of the rules from the book *The House of God*: 'They can always hurt you more.'

'Sorry, I'll get right on it.'

◆◆◆

Most of you probably know of the popular arcade game Whac-A-Mole. Working a shift in a public hospital is like playing this game all day. The nature of the moles has changed over time, though.

When I started as a house officer on general medicine, our team would be on call once a week. On this day, all patients admitted to hospital under general medicine would become your responsibility, or that of one of the other teams that was on call with you. You spent the rest of the week trying to resolve patients' issues and get the numbers down in preparation for the next onslaught. It was like being on a ship taking on water and trying to bail before the next wave hit.

Everyone tried to achieve the mythical 'project zero', which was to discharge all of your patients. Inevitably, patients you had previously discharged would end up being readmitted and would be transferred back to your team, even if it wasn't a day you were on call. These 'handbacks' would destroy any chance of getting down to reasonable numbers. You might go into a 24-hour on-call period (of which you worked 14 hours yourself: 8 a.m. to 10 p.m.) with around 10 patients, and then admit another 30, which meant you had 40 patients to see the following day.

I often found myself staying until 8 p.m. even on my non on-call days, when we were supposed to work 8 a.m. to 5 p.m. There was no prospect of claiming overtime, because the RMO unit would just tell you wouldn't have needed to stay late if you'd worked more efficiently.

The days were spent trying to keep up with discharge summaries, as everybody in the hospital leaned hard on you to empty beds, as if the shortage of beds would be fixed if only you were a bit more efficient. Your pager would not stop.

'Bed 5 has been waiting for three hours for discharge papers!'

'Bed 11 — the ambulance is waiting to take her to the rest home, need the discharge papers!'

'Bed 1 — got tired of waiting and has left. Pls fax script to pharmacy.'

Of course nobody cracking the whip actually wants to help in the process of discharge documentation and writing scripts. That's way too mind-numbing. Everyone is above that. That task falls to the house officer, the completer of all boring and time-consuming tasks.

At some point someone had the bright idea of creating the discharge lounge. This was a space close to the hospital exit, with comfortable sofas, self-serve coffee and tea and out-of-date tabloid magazines, where patients could be sent to wait for their discharge papers, allowing a bed to be freed up.

This was a great idea in theory, until people lost sight of the initial purpose.

'Hi. Did you get my page about Ms Ho, who has been waiting in the discharge lounge for two hours?'

'I did.'

'Well, are you coming down soon?'

'I have five patients to discharge upstairs first.'

'Okay, it's just that she's been waiting a while.'

'Yes, I understand. There's only one of me, so I'll get to her as soon as I can.'

'Do you think you could prioritise her?'

'Doesn't that defeat the whole purpose of having a discharge lounge?'

'Umm, why?'

'Well the priority is to free up beds on the ward, and let patients wait in comfort in the lounge. I need to focus on the patients who are still in their beds.'

'Ms Ho has been waiting a long time. I'm going to have to submit an incident report if you can't come down in the next five minutes.'

I put down the phone and stood staring through the grimy venetians on the window that looked out onto the ward corridor. A janitor was stroking his mop across the linoleum. I wanted to trade places with him. I just wanted to mop floors and get away from this bullshit.

◆◆◆

After-hours the work became more clinical, because suddenly you became the first port of call for all problems. But there were only two of you rostered to attend to the urgent needs of all the medical patients in the entire hospital. The word 'urgent' is variably defined.

On weekends, as well as attending to patients' 'urgent' needs, you also had to complete tasks left by teams that weren't around: review weekend blood test results, review the patients themselves, and discharge any patients who were ready to go home. We referred to all these tasks and calls as 'jobs'.

One Saturday I started the day with 40 jobs. I took a deep breath, rolled up my sleeves and strode up to the ward, because if you don't get off the starting blocks in good time you are quickly lapped.

I went to see the first patient for review. He still wasn't drinking much fluid, and still looked quite dehydrated.

I determined he needed another day of intravenous fluids and sat down to write a prescription.

'Bleep bleep bleep.'

The on-call phone was a considerable advance over the pager, having an app where jobs were messaged to you by nurses, and you could reply.

'Patient Taylor — family here, requesting update. Ta.'

I messaged back: 'I am the on-call, don't know this patient. I don't have the capacity to update families on the weekend.'

'Please if you could update, the family is very upset and threatening to make a complaint.'

Huffing, I signed off my fluid prescription and headed to the nurses' station on the floor below. Patient notes were strewn around the desk and it took forever to find them. I sat down to read what was going on with patient Taylor, then found the family and told them what I could.

'So why didn't he have the CT scan yesterday?' asked the irate son. 'His doctors said he would.'

'I don't know. I'm only the weekend on-call doctor; I'm sorry I don't know the answer.'

He looked down at the ground, his jaw clenched.

'Well, it's just not good enough, you know?'

'Yes, I understand, sir. I'm very sorry.'

In the 20 minutes this took, another 15 jobs had pinged on the phone.

I scrolled through them, trying to find the most urgent ones, a sickening, sinking feeling in my gut. I was already behind.

Another message. 'Patient heart rate 150, plz review. Thanks.'

'Why the fuck was this put through as only semi-urgent?' I asked aloud.

I jogged back upstairs to find that the patient looked okay. He had missed his usual dose of heart-rate-controlling medication that morning so I gave instructions to administer it and call me back if that didn't help.

'He has a whole bunch of usual meds that haven't been prescribed. Could you prescribe them?' asked the nurse.

'Sure.'

I looked at his medication list. Three of them were quite important so I signed off on them. The rest were non-urgent and could wait a couple of days until the regular team were back on. I was about to head off to another patient review when the phone buzzed again.

'Patient requesting his usual statin to be prescribed.'

I texted back.

'Not an after-hours job.'

'This is a 24-hour service, doctor,' was the message back.

Nothing happens if you miss your cholesterol medication for a couple of days. I deleted the job.

'Right, time to see Ms Kumar.'

A message came up in red on the phone.

'Patient found unconscious, GCS 8.'

Okay, this was urgent. I called the nurse and asked them to put out an emergency call. Then I sprinted off to the first-floor ward and arrived to find the emergency response team already attending to the patient. He had low blood sugar, and came right with some intravenous sugar. It took about 20 minutes to sort him out.

'Right, Ivor, do you mind reviewing this guy in about an hour?'

I nodded. Another job to add to the list.

By this time my list had ballooned to 60 jobs. I started to feel a squirm in my stomach and a cool sweat forming on my chest.

After I'd seen Ms Kumar another job popped up.

'Patient has chest drain, due 12-hourly alteplase.'

A chest drain is a tube that passes through the ribs and sits in the chest cavity, draining fluid or infection. If the material in the chest cavity is very thick, a medication called alteplase can be used to loosen it up and allow it to drain more freely. It can, however, cause serious bleeding.

I found the nurse in the medication room.

'I've got them ready for you.' She slapped a kidney dish on the bench.

'Thanks. Hey, how do I mix this up?'

She turned and smiled.

'Well, you just take 20 ml of saline and use it to reconstitute the powder. Then once you've mixed it, take half of that and mix it with another 30 ml of saline.'

'Right, reconstitute with 20 ml, half, then 30 ml . . .' I mumbled. 'Can you do it for me?'

'Sorry, sweety, I'm not allowed.'

She could have done it with her hands tied behind her back, as nurses reconstituted and drew up medications every day. House officers, on the other hand, never did this, yet were expected to draw up this particular medication because of its serious potential side-effects. In some guideline writer's mind it made complete sense to delegate the most dangerous drugs to the person with the least experience.

At least I knew that powder had to be dissolved in saline first before it could be drawn up. I had seen one colleague attempt to draw the powder up directly through the needle and syringe.

I read and re-read the information booklet that came with the drug.

'All right, reconstituting the powder,' I said with more confidence than I felt. I injected 20 ml of saline into the glass vial with the powder. It didn't mix very well. Then I mistakenly let go of the pressure on the syringe and all my saline sucked back up into the syringe, leaving a gloopy mess at the bottom of the vial.

'Try shaking it as you inject the saline, to help the powder to mix,' said a nearby nurse.

'Shake. Right, thanks!'

She looked down at her meds and shook her head with a gentle smile. My collar started to feel very tight.

I tried again and it mixed better. But the needle didn't quite reach into the recess of the vial and some medication was left in there after I pulled it back into my syringe. I went to inject and try sucking it all back up again, but the needle had by now come half out of the rubber stopper. As I pushed on the plunger of the syringe, alteplase pissed into the air and all over my face, the bench and the floor.

Tail between my legs, I went to find the nurse and asked her for another vial. Things went better the second time.

I went to the patient. His chest drain had a three-way valve on one of the connections, allowing you to close off the drainage tube or inject stuff into it.

I spun the valve around and opened the injection port. I looked to the patient.

'This may feel funny for a little bit.'

He nodded.

I injected the alteplase into the drain.

'Shit, shit, shit,' I murmured to myself.

'What did you say, Doctor?'

'Oh nothing, don't worry. I just need to go and get some more medication.'

I had spun the valve 90 degrees further than I should have, and all the medication I had injected had just drained straight back out of the patient and into the collection chamber at the end of the tube.

I went to draw up my third vial of alteplase.

By the time this was all done, the job list had ballooned to 73. I started scrolling through the messages and didn't know where to start. I couldn't even finish reading them all because new ones would pop up and take me to the top of the page again.

'Dr, patient needs laxatives.'

'Hi Dr, patient found on the floor of bathroom.'

'Patient IV line removed as it was 3 days old, needs new IV line, ta.'

'Hi Doctor, patient would like to talk to you about her medication, is refusing antibiotics, is being treated for pneumonia, thanks.'

'Ward 68 here, patient had a portable fan fall off the shelf and hit her on the head. Complaining of headache, please review.'

'Please review, patient complaining of nausea, already given ondansetron, metoclopramide, cyclizine, dexamethasone and Scopoderm, no effect.'

'Hello doctor, urgent, patient threatening to leave against medical advice, please come to review. Ta!'

I started to feel really hot. My head was swimming and I could feel my stomach acid reaching with both hands for the sides of my gullet. I found the sluice room and sat down, fanning myself with my hands as I stared into space. A mirage formed in the distance. I saw myself throwing the on-call phone into the patient toilet and walking away. The image floated like a cloud, spreading out between the sterile walls of the corridor, its thin wisps reaching out and caressing my face.

I shook myself from my daydream, pushed down the nausea, got up and marched on. The lost traveller knows that once they start seeing mirages, lying down for a rest means death. The only way to survive is to push through the exhaustion and try to make it out of the desert.

I didn't sit down, other than to write notes, until 4 p.m. My job list peaked at triple figures. By 10 p.m. it was down to 20.

◆◆◆

Things have changed at my old hospital in the past 10 years, and there are now more than double the number of on-call house officers. The on-call system works differently, too, with admissions being more evenly spread between more teams over more days. A hospital that was previously a first-year doctor's last choice is now considered cushy and sought after.

In fact the rest of us gripe that house officers these days have it too easy. They don't get as much experience as we did, and they will never know the feeling of being waterboarded with jobs. We used to do seven night shifts in a row; now three or four is the norm.

I'm fully aware of the irony that when we went on strike in our first year, fighting for the right to not have to work 12 days without break, the older doctors said the same thing about us. We had it too easy, according to them. How we hated them for being so out of touch and thinking that just because they endured abusive working conditions, we should too.

Every generation wants to wear its formative experiences as a badge of honour.

◆◆◆

However, despite improvements in working conditions for new graduates, things generally, and for all the other grades of hospital doctor, are worse than ever.

A few months ago I was called down to the ED at 2 a.m. to review a sick child who probably needed to be admitted to the ICU. She had severe asthma and wasn't responding to the usual treatments.

In the paediatric resus bay I found my colleague Chloe hunched over a preschooler, listening to her lungs.

One of the cool things about working in the hospital system — and there aren't many — is that after a while your old friends and acquaintances start assuming senior positions.

I grinned and nodded my head upwards at her.

'Hey stranger, how's it going?' she asked, beaming back.

'Oh you know, it goes. Yourself?'

She pouted and gestured broadly at the rest of the kids' emergency department, every last cubicle packed with waiting parents and children.

'Ah, yes, of course, of course. So what's going on here?'

'Well, this four-year-old has frequent admissions to ED with asthma, started on montelukast a few months ago. Runny nose last couple of days, became short of breath this evening, having 20-minute inhalers at home. Has come into ED with severe work of breathing, has gone down the IV therapy algorithm with magnesium, salbutamol, aminophylline. A bit better since then but still struggling.'

I looked over at the child. She was leaned back against her mother, bug-eyed and still, other than her chest which was heaving to and fro. A quiet child is welcome news when it's well, not so much when it's ill.

'Okay, we'll get a bed ready up on the ICU and try a bit of CPAP [a special oxygen mask that provides extra pressure to help inflate the lungs] and see if that helps.'

'Perfect.'

We moved away from the bed, and I furrowed my brow as I realised that something didn't feel right about the whole situation.

'Hang on,' I said to Chloe. 'Why are you here at 2 a.m.? Where's your registrar? Did they ask you to come in?'

Chloe had been a specialist paediatrician for two years and would be expected to be on call from home after-hours while a paediatric registrar manned the fort.

She leaned her head back and laughed at the ceiling.

'Keep up, mate! Half of our registrar positions are unfilled this year. We're all having to fill in the gaps. Patrick's actually the one on call, I'm just the registrar tonight.'

'What the fuck? How does that even happen?'

She shrugged. 'Nobody wants to do paeds. Maybe they've all buggered off overseas, who knows? It's not just this hospital.'

'But that's bullshit. You didn't do all that training to be stuck here in the middle of the night over a decade later.'

She raised her eyebrows at me.

'I'm not finished yet,' I replied to the silent question.

She shrugged.

'It is what it is, Ivor. Somebody's gotta do it.'

'It's a paeds thing. You won't see the adult physicians filling in for their registrars. Or surgeons.'

'Well, people care more if a baby dies than a granny.'

◆◆◆

In fact adult medicine is going through the same crisis. When I finished my rotation in general medicine in the first part of 2023, the rotation after mine had failed to fill half of its registrar positions. It's the same across many hospitals, and continued in 2024. Some teams were operating without a registrar at all.

Registrars are supposed to be the backbone of the team: the perfect crossover of ability and availability. They have the experience to sort out problems that the house officers might struggle with, yet the lack of seniority to escape the coalface.

On my last day of being a registrar in the adult medical service I walked into the hospital with a bounce. I had only nine hours of servitude left, and there were only so many ways I could be hurt in that time.

My colleague who had been on nights looked at me as if I was a cruise ship that had come across him stranded in the middle of the Atlantic. His sallow face brightened as he thrust the on-call phone and pager towards me.

'Take them,' he said.

I nodded in understanding.

'One of the other admitting registrars has called in sick, and they've pulled the other one to cover a gap in cardiology, so it's just you. And a lot of patients came in at 7 a.m., so there's already five waiting. Good news is they've said we no longer need to go to medical emergency calls in ED.'

'How come?'

He shrugged. 'Not enough of us to go around. Anyway, see ya!'

He shot out of there like the Roadrunner. Did an AMF-YOYO.

Adios, motherfucker, you're on your own.

I went and looked at the board.

Chest pain, collapse, stroke, chest pain, collapse.

The problem with starting the day with patients already waiting is that the floodgates open early in the morning and five can quickly become 15.

Should I try and crank through as many patients as possible, with the risk of missing something? Or should I devote the time required to each patient, and thereby also risk missing something by not getting to it in time?

I decided it didn't really matter because I was screwed either way.

The first patient was a delightful chap of 95, sitting in a plastic chair in an ED cubicle with two other elderly men beside him.

'Which one of you is Elwin?'

'That'd be me.'

'And these are your . . . relatives?'

One of the others piped up.

'No relation. We're all patients. They just shoved us all in here cos they didn't have nowhere else.'

'Oh. Okay.'

So much for patient privacy.

'Can you walk okay, Elwin? Why don't we find somewhere private to talk?'

We walked down the corridor but every cubicle was occupied, some clearly with multiple patients. We settled for a supply closet at the end of the hall.

'It's feeling mighty tight in my chest right now, Doctor,' he said as I closed the door behind us.

'Is that the reason you've come?'

He nodded as he caught his breath.

'Do you feel that tightness anywhere else?'

'Yeah, in my neck. Feel a bit sick too.'

It's not often a patient gives you a textbook description of angina.

I proceeded to examine him standing up, fully clothed, and surrounded by mops.

My phone rang.

'Excuse me.'

I stepped outside and took the call.

'Hey, how are you? I'm just calling to refer you this 80-year-old. Family dropped her off this morning saying she's more confused than normal.'

'More than normal?'

'Yeah, she's got Alzheimer's. Anyway, can't find much on examination, bloods look okay, have done a screen for infection which is negative, head scan which is normal, but obviously she'll need to come your way for further work-up.'

'What else is there to work up? If it's all normal why can't the family just take her back home?'

'Well, she's not at her baseline. Also the family have left.'

'What do you mean left? Where have they left to?!'

'They're going out of town for the weekend, back Monday.'

There was the kicker. The classic granny dump.

'So the patient can't give any history, the family are not around to tell us anything, and the diagnosis is that she needs a new family?'

'That's about it. Look, I don't like calling you about this any more than you like taking the call, but it is what it is. I don't have a lot of time, I've got patients coming out my eyeballs here, so I'm gonna leave this with you, all right? She won't be a lot of work — just tuck her in and you can discharge her on Monday.'

I'll be making a report to Age Concern is what I'll be doing, I thought.

No sooner had I stepped back into the supply closet than the phone rang again.

'Hello?'

I looked over to Elwin to mouth an apology but he was busying himself with inspecting the cleaning supplies.

It was a GP from an urgent care centre. 'Listen, I just want to get some advice. I've got this patient who clinically has a DVT [blood clot in the leg], but obviously tomorrow's the weekend, and she doesn't want to wait around in hospital all weekend for an ultrasound scan on Monday. What do you think is the likelihood of her being able to get a scan today?'

'I don't really know. I don't control the radiology lists, but things are pretty hectic today. I would say the chances are probably low, but we can try.'

'Mmm, yeah, okay. Well, what are the chances of getting it over the weekend if she goes in and doesn't get it today?'

'I've never seen a DVT scan get done over the weekend.'

I looked over at Elwin and rolled my eyes, shaking my head from side to side to show I hadn't forgotten about him.

'Yeah, thought so. I guess I'll just have to give her blood thinners over the weekend. But it's annoying not to be able to get an urgent scan in this situation.'

'Yup, well, we're just serving fries at Café Health New Zealand; no salt, no pepper, no ketchup.'

She laughed.

I went back to the supply closet and told Elwin he might need an angiogram to look for blockages in his heart vessels, although at his age it might be best to try him on some anti-angina medications first and see how he went. But his symptoms were quite severe, so he could have a large blockage that might not respond to medication. According to his blood tests his angina had not progressed to a full-on heart attack. I decided we would admit him overnight for observation and ask a cardiologist to see him.

Not wanting to provoke further angina in the meantime, I called for an orderly and a wheelchair to return him to his crowded cubicle.

As I walked back through the long rectangular space that was the main part of the ED, the text alert on my phone went off.

'My mother's foot hurts and she can't walk,' it read.

'Fuck me,' I said aloud to myself. How had this person got the on-call number?

I actually felt some sympathy for this stranger. They were just trying to do their best for a parent. But I couldn't help. Just as I didn't answer the landline when it rang next to me at the nurses' station. Just as I didn't help patients to the toilet or go and grab their lunch for them. Not because I'm an arsehole but because you can't be the solution to every problem, even if each solution takes just a minute. You have to look after yourself because no one else will. Expose yourself too much, and the system will strip every last bit of flesh you have.

Then my personal phone alert went off.

'Hospital having unexpected surge today, at 110% capacity, please remember to discharge all patients as early as possible.'

I contemplated that the managers needed to go back to primary school to learn about percentages, not to mention basic English.

'You can't be at over 100 per cent capacity,' I had argued to one of them a few weeks earlier, over after-work drinks.

'Yes you can. You have a capacity; and then you go over it!'

'Yes, but then that becomes your new capacity. Capacity remains at 100 per cent. What you're talking about is the capacity you want, relative to the capacity you have. There's a different word for that.'

'Okay then, Mr Shakespeare, what is it?'

'Fiction.'

He tightened his lips into an unyielding line and stared at me.

I was not about to let up.

'Furthermore,' I said, pointing my finger up in the air as if I was standing at a lectern, 'something ceases to be unexpected when it starts happening every day.'

He was still stuck on the numbers. 'Rugby players always talk about having given 110 per cent at the end of the game.'

'Well, they've taken a few too many knocks to the head, haven't they?'

◆◆◆

The on-call phone rang again.

'Doctor, we need you urgently on the maternity ward!'

'Umm, okay. Have you put out an emergency call?'

'What? No, just come to Room 17, quickly!'

'Okay I will, but put out a call please.'

I followed my rule of never running to an emergency, but decided a speed walk was acceptable in this situation.

When I arrived on the maternity ward, the nurse furrowed her brows and looked up and down at my white shirt with red lapels and creased black pants.

'Who are you?'

'You called me just a minute ago. What's the matter? Pulmonary embolism? Peripartum cardiomyopathy?'

She recoiled her head and shoulders even further back.

'No . . . no. She's ready to deliver, doctor. What's your name, by the way? I've never seen you before.'

My shoulders sagged. The howling from behind the curtain made sense now.

'I think there's been a misunderstanding,' I said. 'Who did you think you were calling?'

'The obstetric registrar.'

'Right, well, you got put through to the wrong phone. I'm the medical registrar.'

She opened her mouth and tilted her head back.

'Ahh.'

'I mean, I could try and deliver this baby. But it's been 10 years since I delivered a baby, and that one had a post-partum haemorrhage, so maybe it's not the best idea.'

I returned to the admissions unit hub and looked over the patient waiting list. Two more patients had been added. And I had missed two calls.

Over the next couple of hours I saw six patients and took six more referrals. My net progress was stationary. 'Just keep your head above water,' I repeated to myself.

June was the next patient waiting to be seen. She was 92 years old and lived in the private hospital wing of the nearest residential care facility. She had been sent to hospital because the care-home staff noticed she was breathing funny. June was bedridden from a previous stroke and spent her days either in bed or sitting in a chair, into which she had to be hoisted.

June also could not speak. She had carers who did

everything for her, including changing her nappies. She was doubly incontinent.

I came into the ED cubicle to find her lying in bed and staring up at the ceiling. The bed was too short for her, and one leg was drooping down over the edge. Her body was pointed one way across the bed and her head was angled the other way, so that she looked like a hockey stick. The sheets had half fallen off her. The rest of the room was empty.

'Hi June, I'm Ivor, one of the doctors.'

I stroked her hand to let her know I was there.

She continued staring up at the ceiling and mumbled. 'Bhaa, ahh, ahh, bhaa.'

'I know, dear, I know.'

I pulled on the under-sheet to straighten her out as best I could, and lifted her wayward leg back onto the bed. I examined her, going fishing for some abnormality. All I could find was that she had a fever and was breathing fast. Her breathing sounded gurgly, but I had no idea what it sounded like normally. She was skin and bone, and her skin was dry and cracked. The most likely diagnosis was that she had pneumonia. If you spend your days lying in bed, nasty infection-causing bugs tend to settle in your lungs.

I went back to the ED fishbowl and started rifling through her notes.

I rang her next of kin, her son, to try to get more information but my call went to voicemail.

Next I called the rest home. It took 11 minutes to reach a nurse. (I counted.)

'Are you the nurse looking after June? I'm one of the doctors at the hospital.'

'I was around this morning when the ambulance came to pick her up.'

'Okay great, well, I was hoping you could tell me a bit more about what happened.'

'Well, she had been fine up until last night—'

'Sorry, when you say "fine" — um, she's normally non-verbal, correct? Does she normally make random sounds?'

'She doesn't speak, and she only tends to make a lot of sounds when she's unwell. That's how we knew something was off last night.'

'Okay, sorry to interrupt. Please continue.'

'Well, so she was doing that last night, and then this morning we noticed she was breathing harder than normal, and she seemed a bit shaky, and then she had a really high temperature. That's when we called an ambulance.'

'Is her breathing normally gurgly?'

'No, that's not normal for her.'

'Okay . . . wait what's this?'

I had been flicking through photocopied notes from the rest home during the conversation. One was titled 'Advance Care Planning.' In a very serious font, it outlined that June did *not* wish to be readmitted to hospital anymore, and that if she became ill, she should be managed at the facility. It was dated several years ago, when she had first moved to the facility and was still able to communicate, and was signed by June herself.

I told the nurse what I had found.

'Oh, yes, that's her advance care plan.'

'Yes.'

There was an uncomfortable silence.

'You still there?'

'Yes, yes.'

'So if she has an advance care plan, why didn't you, um, follow it?'

I was trying to be delicate.

'Because she seemed very unwell. I don't think we could manage her here like that. And last time she got unwell her family said they still wanted her admitted to hospital.'

'Actually the family cannot override her directive. Do you have an on-call GP for situations like this?'

'Yes, but they're not available until the end of the week. Our local GP practice is too busy and they've had to cut back their availability. Look, *Doctor*, I've been doing this for 20 years. Don't talk to me like I'm stupid. I know what an advance care directive means. I know that the most dignified thing would be that she dies in the rest home in peace with some medications to make her comfortable. But if the family wants her to go to hospital and get poked and prodded with needles, left alone because there's not enough nurses to take care of all the patients, become more confused and then get diarrhoea from the antibiotics you are no doubt going to give her, well it's not my arse that's going to stand in the way and get handed a complaint when we can't even get a doctor here to support us.'

Wow. I felt a wave of contrition. 'I'm sorry. I know.'

After I put down the phone I sat for a while with my head in my hands.

◆◆◆

By lunchtime I had received reinforcements. At this stage we were losing the beachhead and had been pushed all the way back to the shoreline. Twelve patients were waiting to be seen. I went and had lunch. Put on your own oxygen mask first.

I spent the afternoon seeing patients in corridors. I argued with some surgical doctors about whether a patient with pancreatitis should be admitted under medicine or surgery. I got berated by a family for leaving them waiting so long. I rushed back and forth to attend to emergencies on the ward and acute strokes in the emergency department. I answered endless phone calls, including a period of time where back-to-back calls had me on the phone for 25 minutes straight.

The last patient of the day told me I was an idiot for telling him his breathing was getting worse because of his emphysema and desire to keep smoking rather than because of the Covid vaccine, and asked me how much Big Pharma had paid me to participate in a genocide. I opened my mouth to inform him that if I wanted to make a living off shilling pharmaceuticals, standing here listening to his moronic statements would be the first employment I would drop, but seeing as how I didn't have this lucrative career to fall back on, I thought better of it.

By evening handover I was walking around with phone in outstretched hands, like a zombie, looking for the first available person to hand off to.

'AMF-YOYO,' I whispered to myself as I handed the flaming torch to Amy. Half of the evening rota was unfilled and there were now 20 patients waiting to be seen.

I laughed as I made a beeline for the door. I thought of basketball. Back when Kobe Bryant was still alive and dominating the NBA he came across an elite defender by the name of Shane Battier. Battier had studied years' worth of tapes of Kobe's play. He knew exactly how often he would dribble with his left or his right hand. He knew Kobe's shooting percentages at each location on the court. He knew exactly which teammates Kobe was likely to pass to and at which point in the game. He knew the man's inclinations, thoughts and flaws perhaps better than Kobe himself.

He defended Kobe during a crucial playoff game, and played a blinder of a defence, yet Kobe scored 40 points on him and won the game. In the post-match interview Battier just laughed, because what else could he do?

When you work your arse off and leave after every shift exhausted, yet you hand over 20 waiting patients to your colleagues, you feel like crap. What are you supposed to do other than laugh? When constantly seeing bad shit happen that you cannot control, most hospital doctors do one of three things. Some experience all the emotions fully. They often don't last long before they burn out. Some become arseholes who let nothing in. Nobody likes these people. Most of us let the emotions in, but protect ourselves against the full impact by dulling the edge of the blade that they travel on.

The best 'dulling agent' is laughter. We don't laugh and make jokes because we think the things that happen to people are funny. It is precisely because they are not funny that we need to find a way to make them so. This is the strategy that results in the most longevity for your career.

On my way out I walked past Jackie, one of the first-year registrars. Jackie was on the phone to one of the ED specialists.

'Look, I really don't think this patient needs to come into hospital. We've already got 20 patients waiting to be seen. Why don't you just increase her dose of furosemide and get her to follow up with her GP in a couple of days.'

I stopped and smiled, remembering the days when I too thought it was my responsibility to be a brick wall, and guard the system against the consequences of its own underinvestment. One of the specialists had told me: 'Ivor, the truth is that nobody is calling to ask your opinion. On the other end of the line you have a specialist in emergency medicine, who has far more training and experience than you. If they think the patient needs to be admitted, then the patient is getting admitted. It's just a courtesy call, really. The sooner you realise you're just a cog, here to do any work that comes your way, the sooner you'll stop wasting your time arguing with people, and the more at peace you will be.'

I gave Jackie the same advice.

◆◆◆

So why are we short so many registrars? Are junior doctors chasing the coastal big-city dream right across the ditch in Australia, with better money and more affordable living? Certainly that is the word on the ground.

As fun as such anecdotes are, it is necessary to look at the data, and this has not always been obliging. The Medical Council keeps track of New Zealand-trained doctor retention — by each postgraduate year, and grouped by graduation date into five-year blocks. The problem is that there is a natural lag in the data, which makes it hard to know what is going on at the moment. For example, the 2021–25 cohort only has data available up to postgraduate year 3, and less of it. And it is at about postgraduate year 3 that people start leaving, because there are more opportunities at this level.

However, the 2024 workforce report clearly shows for the first time a downturn in doctor retention, when for most of the time since 2005 it had been improving. The talk on the street is right. We are not competitive with the career opportunities and pay overseas (Australia and elsewhere).

But with every move there is both a push and a pull. Who would want to work day in and day out at the job

I have just been describing? The dirty face of bed-block and lack of physical resources staring at you every day is further tipping personal decisions in favour of getting the hell out of Dodge.

As we have seen, the problem does not lie in a lack of doctors graduating from medical school. The workforce data also show that we are training more than enough doctors to keep up with population growth. Every year since I graduated, and probably a lot longer than that, New Zealand has graduated more doctors than there are jobs for them. It would also be difficult to further increase medical school numbers without diluting medical students' on-the-job experience. Hospital doctors are not paid or given protected time to teach medical students on placement; it is all voluntary.

Needless to say, politicians' solution of building a new medical school in Waikato is a fart in the wind.

The problem is the shortage of registrars — junior doctors at least three years out from graduation. (We're short of specialists too, but we'll talk about that later.) And it's not just that the registrars are leaving for Australia. A turning point occurred after the strike for safer rosters, in which I took part, in 2016. Following this, the maximum days that could be worked consecutively dropped from 12 to 10, and the maximum nights went from 7 to 4. We now needed more registrars to do the same amount of work.

The system was able to stay afloat for a while by convincing its most junior cogs that they were pursuing more than just a career; that this was something to which they should devote themselves to the exclusion of everything else. It squeezed every last drop of blood, sweat and tears out of them. When doctors finally started saying, 'No more,' the cracks began to show.

Specialties like medicine, ED and paediatrics tend to be more affected by registrar shortages than surgical specialties. In this case, for example, many surgical departments did not abide by the new roster restrictions. Their registrars preferred to work more and get paid more, and this led to the formation of a splinter union.

At the same time, the increasingly complex services needed to meet the needs of our ageing population have resulted in new registrar positions being created in subspecialty departments such as respiratory, gastroenterology and infectious diseases, and these have soaked up doctors from the general medicine registrar pool. These jobs are far more appealing because they don't have to deal with every problem that comes through the front door, pulling you every which way until you want to pull your hair out. Paediatrics and emergency medicine have the same 'front-door syndrome'.

As doctors enter their registrar years, burnt out by a few years on a hospital roster, they look around and see better offers, so many opt to pursue them. This has made the system reliant on international medical graduates to come in and fill the gaps. And yet in recent years the number of foreign doctors employed as registrars has started to drop.

In short, while there is no shortage of house officers

in hospitals, there are nowhere near enough registrars for the amount of work. How do we address this problem?

Pay that competes with salaries overseas is an obvious one. But if registrars felt valued in a non-monetary sense, and didn't spend their days living in the twilight zone in an underfunded system, that would be a good start too. It would help a lot if there were more specialist training positions.

And if we as a society had realistic expectations about what a hospital can and cannot achieve for patients, so that health services in the community could relieve some of the burden on hospitals, that would be the icing on the cake. Maybe the country could retain more of the skilled practitioners we invest in producing and we would all be better off.

10.

WAITING FOR GODOT

When I was a medical student I was sent to take a case history from a patient who had come in with abdominal pain. I spent an hour exploring his symptoms, his medical history, his alcohol intake and his sex life. On the latter two counts, he led a much more exciting life than I did.

I went on to express my sympathies for the distress he was experiencing, like a good little student doing as he was taught, and I noticed his weathered countenance expressing increasing discomfort as I talked. There was something about the bushy sideburns, muddy boots and flannel shirt that told me that the standard-issue med school communication technique might not work on him. I considered addressing smoking cessation but thought better of it.

After about an hour I realised I should get back to the specialist who was supervising me, lest she got worried and filed a missing person's report. I said goodbye to my patient and went and sat in the office, collating my rag-tag scribbles into some structured summary.

Dr Xena was sitting at a computer in the admissions unit hub sipping on a latte. She had on a poufy frock that made it impossible for anyone to pass her in a corridor and was so bright yellow you almost needed sunglasses. Purple stockings completed the look.

She pulled her horn-rimmed glasses down her nose to look at me as I entered.

'Ah, the prodigal son returns! I was about to send out a search party. Come and sit, and tell me what you've found.'

She pulled up a chair and patted it enthusiastically.

I swallowed and began.

'So, the patient is a 60-year-old male who—'

Her phone rang.

'Sorry. One second.'

'Yes, hello Mark . . . No, I told the patient to come at 2 p.m. He's here now? . . . Well, that's just not really . . . No, I'm in the middle of something . . . okay, well, they'll just have to wait . . . yes, you can tell them that . . . okay, ciao.'

She turned back to me.

'Sorry about that, I just—'

The phone rang again.

She clenched her jaw, which brought out dimples at the corners of her mouth.

'Hello, it's Dr Xena. Okay, tell me about the patient . . . Is he on blood thinners? . . . When did he last eat? . . . Hmm, any comorbidities? Okay, yes, can you put through an electronic request? Okay, ciao.'

She turned to face me again and huffed.

'So. The patient is a 60-year-old—'

Ring, ring.

She threw her head back in exasperation. This time she had to go. She fixed me with her gaze. 'Look, I'm so sorry, I'll be back in about 10 minutes and we can go over your case presentation then, okay?'

'Yes, yes, no problem, I'll sit here and practise.'

When she came back half an hour later, hair slightly frizzled, I was sitting in the exact same spot. I had spent the time observing the foot traffic in and out of the admissions hub, eyes glazed over in some hazy fog of inertia that made it hard to even open my mouth now and make words. Perhaps as a result, what did come out was a little disinhibited.

'It seems to me that 50 per cent of a medical student's day is spent waiting.'

She narrowed her eyes, looked me up and down, then let out an icy laugh.

'Honey, you think that stops as you get more senior? Ha! No, you just have to wait on different things. Half my work life is spent waiting for something or someone. Half my actual life is spent waiting for something or someone. You're gonna have to get used to it.'

I nodded.

'There's a good book about it,' she continued. 'Have you ever read Samuel Beckett's play *Waiting for Godot*?'

I shook my head.

'I recommend it. It's all about how life is about waiting.'

◆◆◆

I vividly remember waiting for Covid-19. I worked in the ICU during the pandemic. Like everyone else, we heard mutterings about a deadly virus in China. People were being admitted to intensive care, and they were dying.

We sprang quickly into the classic fear response that we later came to despise in others: denial. 'It's overblown. It's just happening in China. It will be like all the pandemics over the years that never came to anything. It will all settle down.'

Then cases started appearing in Japan, Thailand and South Korea. Still a world and a culture away from us, though. Then people started dying in Italy and the United States. This was the Western world, so now we started to pay attention. Despite the geographical distance, it became impossible to deny the inevitable now, as least for people who are swayed by logic and evidence.

Inevitably, cases started to appear in New Zealand. We closed our borders. We locked down. And then we waited.

We waited for sick patients to start hitting hospitals. We had no idea whether it would be a small stream, easily dammed with a few logs of wood, or a tsunami, with no safe option but getting to high ground, leaving people in body bags in the corridors as had happened in Italy.

We were twitchy. It felt like sitting on death row, but having no clue whether the next morning you would wake up to guards waiting to escort you down that long corridor. New isolation rooms were hastily built, wards restructured, the ICU reconfigured, new protocols developed, and staff drilled with military precision.

As if we were watching a horror film we sat glued to the awful plight of our overseas counterparts. Unidentified patients dying in the corridors, overflowing morgues and mass graves, shortages of ventilators and beds. We shared reports of experimental or theoretical treatments, like hooking up multiple patients to the same ventilator.

We knew the situation could be even worse for us as we had fewer ICU beds and nurses than some other countries had. We knew that if it was the tsunami that was coming, our preparation was nought but a wooden shelter built at sea level.

We became trigger-happy, admitting a lot of 'suspected Covid' cases whose tests came back clear the next day. There was almost a sense of disappointment at these false alarms. The anticipation was killing us. *Just fucking come and do your worst already.*

Lockdown was eerie, with the deserted streets, the 10-minute commute to work that usually took 40, the constant quiet. I imagined dissonant violins playing as the soundtrack to my life most days.

Management informed us that we were not allowed to wear masks unless we were with a patient with confirmed Covid. They removed face-mask dispensers and told nurses and doctors to remove their masks because we didn't want to scare anyone. The occasional colleague had a mask snatched out of their hand. They didn't have enough personal protective equipment (PPE) for everyone. Reality was scary, so they opted to live in fantasy. The PPE they did provide was one-size-fits-all. I am six foot six, and the sleeves of the protective gowns did not quite reach my wrists.

The prevailing wisdom at the beginning was that Covid was only spread by droplets, so a standard surgical mask, like the ones you see on *Shortland Street* or *Grey's Anatomy*, was enough. The more protective N95 masks, which look like something a fibreglass worker might wear, and which protect against finer aerosols, were considered unnecessary.

Of course we were provided with eye protection against droplets, yet our hair remained uncovered. Hair stuck up from our masked and eye-glassed bodies like sticks of broccoli, obviously considered exempt from being able to spread viral particles through its as-yet-undiscovered magical properties.

Soon enough the sick patients started coming in. Intubating a Covid patient is one of the highest-risk procedures for staff. We were drilled in this, with the most experienced intubator doing the job and minimal other staff in the room. All the necessary equipment came in pre-prepared boxes.

The first time, the rest of us stood watching through the glass doors, marvelling at how slick the team was. Boom, bang — the job was done in three minutes. The intubating doctor came out and doffed his PPE like he was taking off his racing suit and gloves having just completed the Formula One. As we dispersed we muttered to each other how well all the preparation had worked out.

I remained behind to prescribe some medications and slipped the medication chart under the door. As I turned to leave, I heard banging on the glass door.

I turned around to see the nurse inside the room staring at me intently. It's disconcerting when all you can see of someone's expression is their eyes.

She slapped her hand to the door. Under it was a note.

'Patient needs an NG tube.'

A nasogastric is a thin tube inserted through the nose that makes its way down to sit in the stomach, where it drains excessive gastric juices and can be used to give medications in someone who is unconscious.

I looked around. It was just me. I found a piece of paper and scribbled a note in reply.

'Didn't they put one in when they intubated?'

She shook her head slowly.

I cursed under my breath and donned my too-short PPE.

A nasogastric insertion is usually easy when a patient is awake. They are able to swallow, which helps guide the nasogastric to where it needs to go. When they are unconscious it is a completely different story. Not only can they not swallow, but the opening to the food-pipe tends to collapse down. The tube itself is thin and flexible and can bend on itself when being pushed. It is one of those procedures that involves as much luck as skill.

On my first attempt I tried to insert it blindly, pushing it through the nose and hoping it would follow the natural curvature of the back of the nose and mouth into the food pipe. But it kept coiling up on itself.

Then I grabbed the curved metal blade used to lift up the tissues at the back of the throat during intubation, trying to lift the tongue so I could see the opening of the food pipe. I could barely make out a small black hole off to the left; I just couldn't get the tube to go into it. I kept trying and trying and trying. PPE doesn't breathe very well and soon I was sticky and damp.

Still I kept at it.

After a while I was grabbed by a strong smell. It was

vicious, sour, and reminded me of stale cabbage. It reached with long grimy fingers and unkempt fingernails into the back of my own throat and scratched at the lining.

I was smelling the patient's breath.

After 45 minutes the nasogastric was finally in place. Almost an hour of standing in front of the open mouth of a Covid patient.

I reflected that perhaps the intubation protocol had not considered all the facets.

◆◆◆

Another Covid case we had was also very sick. They were unconscious and on the ventilator but we were struggling to get oxygen into their lungs. One of the more effective strategies in this situation is a manoeuvre called 'proning'. You could be forgiven for thinking this involves some advanced technology. Perhaps a complex procedure that requires the doctor's utmost concentration and not too many coffees beforehand. Nope. Proning means lying the patient on their front. After 50 years of intensive care research, one of our most effective treatments is flipping someone over like a rotisserie chicken. It works by helping to redistribute the blood flow in the lungs, and improving the function of the diaphragm, your most important breathing muscle.

If you've ever tried to flip over your somnolent snoring partner in the middle of the night, you'll appreciate that it is not a one-person job.

I stood at the head of the bed holding on to the breathing tube so it wouldn't fall out as we turned.

In front of me were five nurses, three on one side of the patient and two on the other. We were talking among ourselves.

'All right, so on three, we'll move over to the left side of the bed.'

'Over here?'

'No, the other left.'

'Who's going to watch the lines?'

'I can do that.'

'Where did you put the pillows?'

'They're down . . . wait, I don't know . . . oh yes, they're over here.'

'Okay, ready on three . . . one, two, three.'

'Ughh.'

We heaved the patient like a sandbag over to the edge of the bed.

'Phew. Okay, so now we'll flip 90 degrees, then Sam, you put the pillows down, and then on three again we'll lower onto the pillows.'

'Okay, ready on three . . . one, two, three.'

There was a loud pop and a sudden sound like a vacuum cleaner. Something wet hit my bare neck between my gown and mask.

The ventilator tubing had disconnected from the breathing tube while we were turning the patient over. Condensation mixed with patient secretions had sprayed out and misted my neck like some sort of virus-laden aftershave. I grimaced as I quickly reconnected the tubing.

Everyone was staring at me in shock.

'All right,' I said, 'let's carry on. Down with the pillows and then let's lower the patient onto their front.'

I pushed away the rising fear in my chest, pretending this hadn't just happened.

We went again on the count of three. The patient was successfully prone.

'We've lost end tidal,' said one of the nurses with a hint of panic.

The end tidal is a monitor that tells you whether the patient is still getting oxygen from the ventilator. A loss of end tidal means they are not.

I looked around. All the connections were secure. The pressures on the ventilator screen were super-high — as if the revs on your car are in the red zone but the car ain't moving.

There was one obvious explanation. Taking a deep breath, I reached into the patient's mouth with a hooked finger and felt along the breathing tube. I found the spot where, during turning, the plastic tube had been pushed up against the patient's teeth and had kinked, blocking the tube. I wiggled it from side to side to pull it off the teeth and straighten out the kink.

'End tidals back!' said the nurse.

I pulled out my finger and looked at my gloved hand. The rosy pad of my finger was staring back at me through the hole the patient's teeth had made in the glove.

I went home, showered, flicked on the telly, and

waited for my inevitable death. To make myself feel better I remembered an old-school anaesthetist I had worked with who never wore gloves.

'The problem with gloves,' he said, 'is that you get complacent. People think gloves will protect you, but they really don't. There are microscopic holes in the gloves that allows germs to pass through.'

He enlightened me about this one time as I stood watching him try to get a difficult intravenous line into a patient. He paused and turned to look at me.

'You wouldn't use a glove as a condom, now would you?'

He turned back to the unconscious patient and continued silently prodding them with a needle, as if there could be no possible challenge to this unassailable logic.

One of the techs piped up.

'You would if you had a hand-shaped penis!'

◆◆◆

After some time, people started accepting that Covid was spread by aerosols, and N95 masks became more widely used. These masks are designed to fit tightly. Since people have different-shaped faces, you need to undergo mask fit-testing to determine what type of mask fits you best.

There was initially a flaccid attempt by the powers that be to fit-test healthcare staff, but after a few weeks it all became too hard. We received an email that read:

> We have decided not to participate in any further mask fit testing. The failure rate has been much higher than expected and since we only have access to one type of mask, this has created significant anxiety for people. Also, it is important to realise that a mask alone won't protect you, and we don't want to detract focus from other processes to keep us safe.

In one of those late-night impulses that I perhaps should have slept on, I fired back an irate 'reply all' email:

> I am unhappy with this development . . . Fit-testing of occupational masks is required by the Joint Australia/New Zealand Standard 1715. Ignoring results that are uncomfortable does not seem particularly logical to me. Masks are not everything, but every aspect of PPE should be optimised . . . The logical extreme of this would be to say that no piece of PPE alone is protective, so therefore we shouldn't have PPE at all!

A few weeks later, mask fit-testing was back and new mask types were available.

How can you expect a group of healthcare professionals to support a healthcare system that values their wellbeing so little? The system has relied on goodwill for far too long, and that goodwill is rapidly running out.

All that waiting ended up being a bit anticlimactic. The war ended while we were still in training camp.

◆◆◆

Patients know all about waiting. The vast majority of the day-to-day work is carried out by registrars, not specialists. When you are admitted to hospital, you will almost certainly be seen by a registrar, who will prescribe your initial treatment and order the initial tests. They may send you home, but more likely you will stay overnight, as the specialist won't see you until the morning.

If you are seen in a hospital clinic as an outpatient, there is a good chance it is the registrar who sees you, and they discuss all their patients with the specialist at the end of the clinic day. Even if the registrar is quite capable of solving the problem on their own, at the end of the day, if you are in hospital, you are there for the opinion of the specialist. It is the specialist who carries the burden of responsibility, and who has the power to make difficult or complex decisions. Patients can lie around for quite a while awaiting the attention of the relevant specialist, clogging up hospital beds through no fault of their own.

As a registrar admitting patients to hospital I would often be faced with a quandary. The patient I had just seen likely had nothing particularly wrong with them, or they had something that probably didn't need to be managed in hospital. But in the back of my mind I knew there was always the possibility, if I sent them home, that they might die and end up on the front page of tomorrow's paper.

Even if it is about one in a million, you can never eliminate this possibility. If that happened, the question would not be whether sending them home had been the right thing to do, but 'Why were they sent home without being seen by a specialist?' So the easiest thing to do was to tuck to them in for the night and remove all risk. That also meant I didn't have to waste time typing up their discharge summary and writing a script for their medications when I had other patients rolling in on the waiting board.

It's true that I could have rung the on-call specialist and asked for an opinion over the phone. But it was after 5 p.m. and you didn't bother them for things like this. Not that you would find a policy saying so; it was just one of those tacit rules.

While I have not held back from slagging off surgeons, they are probably the hardest-working group of specialists. Surgeons realise that their job often means coming in after-hours. While this doesn't fill anyone's bosom with a warm fluttery feeling, they accept that it needs to be done. Other specialists are less receptive to being bothered after-hours, or even in-hours.

One time we had just finished our morning rounds. Our specialist was John. He had a black lumberjack's beard and forearms that looked like they could take on a gorilla. His black hair was neatly pushed over to the side with wax and he sported a three-piece suit whose buttons looked as if they might ping off and hit you in the eye at any second.

We sat huddled around the computer desk and John sipped his latte.

'All right, guys, I think we have plans for everyone.'

He turned to look at me, the registrar at the time.

'I've got some admin work to do. You have my number. Please feel free to not call.'

He chuckled. The others followed suit awkwardly. I just smiled and nodded, as I didn't want to argue with someone who looked like he might be a street fighter in his spare time.

The story went that at one point a registrar had called John in the middle of the night to ask about an unwell patient. John was so annoyed at being called when he was on call that he hatched an evil plan.

He waited for the registrar to get home, and at eleven o'clock in the morning, when they were sound asleep after a night shift, he called their mobile.

'Now you know what it's like to get woken up when you're sleeping!'

So, instead of calling him, the other registrars and I would simply clog up the hospital with patients, some of whom probably didn't need to be there.

The next morning the specialist would waltz through and discharge a whole bunch of patients. Or make the complex decisions that would get things moving: more tests or scans, new medications or, in the case of surgeons, whether an operation was required or not.

During the junior doctor strike in 2016 we walked off the job for two days. Many of my colleagues decided to spend the time doing something useful for the community, to show that they were dedicated and to try to retain public goodwill, which tends to wane the longer a strike goes on. They organised blood drives, or gave free first-aid lessons, or planted trees.

I am completely unashamed to say that my mates and I went to the pub.

Over beers we laughed and despaired at the fact that, come Thursday, we were just going to have to work twice as hard to clear a 48-hour backlog. Most of the specialists didn't even know where the discharge summary tab was located. They would have no minions to write their notes for them, or fax their referrals, or answer pages about patients' potassium levels.

The ward I was working on at the time had a small office for the use of junior doctors. My friend Omar sat at a tiny desk right next to the door, and I had my back to the door at my own little desk. The corners of the room were filled up with old journal articles; unused IV lines and other bits of equipment, some still in their packaging; and post-it notes with phone numbers and patient NHIs [National Health Index numbers] scrawled on them.

The office smelt vaguely of mildew. There was no window, and the only source of light was two fluorescent LED strips. One of them didn't work properly and constantly flickered. You tried to avoid spending too much time in the office or else you'd have a migraine by the end of the day.

Omar and I had sent emails about this light on three or four occasions.

'We will endeavour to address this problem as soon as practicable,' came the response.

Dr Kumar was the specialist who would be covering our absence during the strike. We placed bets on how long it would be before the light drove him crazy.

When we arrived back on Thursday, our anxiety about the workload turned to disbelief as we realised that not only was there no backlog, but the hospital was actually emptier than ever.

And the fucking light was fixed. Dr Kumar had had enough after only an hour in the office, and had called the maintenance guy on a number we didn't know existed.

Did patients just stay away from the hospital while the strikes were on? But people don't stop getting sick just because we're not at work, so where were they all? There was no sudden surge afterwards as people who sat on their illnesses finally decided to come and get them seen to, either.

The reality is that specialists simply get things done more efficiently. They are better at triaging referrals from outside the hospital and providing advice that allows patients to be managed in the community. They can go right ahead and discharge patients who don't need to be in hospital. And they can make complex decisions and get tests under way when patients first arrive, at the same time avoiding unnecessary tests. They see the 'big picture' and don't get bogged down by minutiae.

Most importantly, they have the power to make things happen.

Once when I was a house officer we had a patient who had bruised his leg. The trouble was he was on long-term blood thinners because he had a metal heart valve, so he was at risk of forming clots on the valve. The blood sitting in his leg had become infected, and the surgical team had taken him to the operating room to clean out the infected bruise. He had also been seen by the cardiology team, because of his heart valves. All in all, there were three medical teams looking after him, including us.

Blood thinners make you more likely to bleed, so the patient was in a Catch-22. If we restarted his blood thinners too soon he might bleed again from the operation site. If we waited too long, his valve was at risk of forming clots.

The cardiology team came around the morning after his operation. They wrote in his notes: 'We recommend restarting anticoagulation [blood thinners] today.'

The surgical team also came around, and wrote their own note: 'Hold off anticoagulation for now.'

Great. It was my job to call around and clarify what we should do.

I started with the cardiology registrar.

'Hi, this is Ivor with the medical team. Hey, for the patient on Ward 1 you've just seen, you recommended starting anticoagulant today, but the surgeons said not to anticoagulate yet. We're wondering what we should do.'

'He's at high risk of thrombosing [forming a clot on] his valve.'

'Yeah, I realise that, but we have two different recommendations here, so which should we follow?'

'I guess talk to the surgeons and see how high they think the risk of re-bleeding is.'

I hung up and called the surgical doctor, explaining the problem again.

'It's not like I can give you a percentage or something. He's already bled at home while on blood thinners . . . so I would say the chance is not small.'

'Well, we're not really sure what to do here.'

'What do they think the risk of thrombosing the valve is?'

I was back on the phone to the cardiology registrar.

'I can't give you an exact percentage, but it's a mitral valve, so those are the highest risk.'

'Yeah, but the risk is like percentage points per year, right?'

'Maybe. But you've given him reversal [a medication to reverse the effects of the blood thinner] when he first came in, so that increases his risk.'

This went back and forth until my specialist wandered into the office and saw me pulling out my hair.

'Give me the phone,' she said.

She spoke directly to both specialists and sorted the problem in less than five minutes.

'Plan is to start anticoagulation tomorrow. Everybody is in agreement,' she said, then left.

The scenario up to the point where she took the reins happens every day in hospitals. Bureaucratic to and fros that throw large chunks of rust in between the gears of the public health system. Once the true decision-makers get involved, decisions get made and things move forward. It is hard to say no to a specialist.

◆◆◆

I worked through the second lot of strikes in 2019. I was doing a night shift in the ICU.

An emergency call came out from one of the wards at about 2 a.m.

I arrived to find a middle-aged woman with a very swollen face. She was having an allergic reaction to a medication. She was gasping for breath, her skin was bumpy all over (hives) and she was as red as a beetroot. A little squeak was coming out of her with every breath. Her windpipe was so swollen, it was starting to close off.

We hit her hard with treatment. We gave her adrenaline through her drip several times, then eventually started an infusion of adrenaline as well as a nebuliser. We gave her steroids. At first the swelling started to come down and the squeaking went away, but then they started back up again.

I started to sweat and developed an uncomfortable cold feeling in my stomach and fingers and toes. This wasn't working. We needed to get a breathing tube into her before the airway closed off completely. Intubating a patient with a swollen windpipe is difficult and scary because everything looks different when it is swollen.

And it might already be too late to fit a tube through the narrowed airway.

I put out a hospital-wide call for an airway emergency. Then, with a slight tremor, I took a scalpel from the equipment trolley in case I needed to cut through the front of her neck to get into the windpipe that way as a last resort. I got all the other intubating equipment ready.

After a few minutes the doors burst open. I looked up and felt the sense of relief I imagine a soldier must feel on seeing reinforcements coming over the hill.

I had forgotten it was strike day. There were usually three anaesthetic doctors on call at night, and tonight they were all specialists, all experts at intubating. The patient was successfully intubated and rushed to the ICU.

Now, I am not suggesting that specialists should be doing all the frontline work that junior doctors do. You wouldn't retain many specialists if this was your strategy. However, at the moment, specialists are underutilised. They could be better used during regular hours to help expedite decisions and get patients moving through the hospital, making things run a lot more smoothly.

But there are not enough of them. *Every specialty has a major shortage of specialists.* The senior doctors' union estimated in 2024 that there was a 22 per cent shortage of public hospital specialists. Over the years, the *proportion* of the workforce that are non-GP specialists has fluctuated around a steady number, the proportion of GPs has fallen dramatically, and the proportion of registrars has ballooned. (Note that proportions are not to be confused with total numbers.)

The bottleneck in registrars transitioning to specialists is tightening. Partly this is due to the restricted number of training spots. However, in recent years registrar salaries have increased dramatically, while specialist salaries have not. Registrars who have been around for a while and work longer hours may actually take a pay cut to become a specialist, so where is the incentive?

◆◆◆

The other issue, of course, is that specialists are increasingly stuck having to waste their valuable time performing administrative tasks. This is worse now that 'non-frontline' positions have been disestablished by the powers that be.

I once spent six months relieving specialty registrars who were off sick or on leave.

On my first day I was told to report to haematology, a sub-department of the department of medicine. I trudged up to their floor of the hospital. Swinging glass doors sharply demarcated the dusty linoleum of the hospital wards from the slightly less dusty blue carpet of the admin offices. The blue carpet was decorated with oddly patterned swirls, reminiscent of how they decorated bus seats when you were a child. The swirls looked rather as if they had been dropped there by mistake, and made you feel a bit dizzy as you walked on them.

I walked down a long blue corridor towards a faint glint of light in the distance, past signs denoting the sub-departments: respiratory medicine, rheumatology, haematology.

I felt like an airport traveller trying to find his gate.

Only one cubicle was occupied. In it sat Professor Bond, with his back to me. His tousled grey mad-professor hair stuck out like an outcropping above the plastic cubicle dividers.

I coughed gently.

'Excuse me, Professor?'

He continued whatever he was doing.

'Yes, yes, just one second,' he said without looking back.

After about a minute he laid his pen down and swung around on his swivel chair. The tails of his chequered tweed coat ribboned around him as he did.

'Yes? Who are you?'

'My name's Ivor. I'm the relieving haematology registrar this week. I was told to report here.'

He frowned.

'Who are you relieving?'

'Not sure. They don't tell me that.'

'Ah, wait, I remember now. I think we had an email about this actually.'

He turned back around, opened his email and started scrolling through his inbox.

'Come in, sit down, sit down.'

He waved his hand towards a chair.

'Let's see. Looks like James is away this week. Okay, so you'll be doing clinic today.'

I clenched my jaw while trying to hide it. I hated clinic. It was one of the reasons I decided to do intensive care.

'Ever done a haematology clinic before?'

'No.'

'Not to worry, not to worry,' he said. 'I'll tell you everything you need to know.'

He had this interesting habit of looking just past you when he talked to you.

In some specialties the knowledge is fairly easy to pick up if you know enough general medicine. Haematology is not one of them. Most of their patients have blood cancers and are on intricate chemotherapy regimen that you don't really learn about unless you do the job. Or they might be on drugs that are part of a clinical trial.

Many of the cancers are classified by the type of genetic mutation, which is described by a seemingly random combination of numbers and letters. The numbers and letters portend either a fair or a poor prognosis.

'So, your first patient will be lovely Fiona. She's just started second-line treatment for myeloma.' He rattled off the names of some drugs I had never heard of. 'This is just a catch-up to see how she's going. So, you know, just ask her about the common side-effects, to see if we need to make any dose reductions.'

'Any side-effects in particular? I'm not really familiar with these drugs.'

'You know, just the common ones.'

'Right. And how bad does it need to be before we consider dropping the dose?'

'It depends on the side-effect and which drug is most likely to be causing it.'

'I see.' I didn't.

'Just call me after the clinic to discuss. I have to do all the chemo scripts anyway. Right, next we have a new patient. I haven't met her before, obviously, but she's had a biopsy of some enlarging nodes in her neck and it's come back with diffuse large B-cell [a type of non-Hodgkin's lymphoma]. We'll plan to treat her with R-CHOP [a type of chemo regimen]. So you just have to break the news to her, and then explain what the treatment will involve.'

I stared back at him until he started to look a little unnerved.

'You've broken bad news before, right?'

'Yes, but usually I tell patients the cancer expert will come and talk to them and answer detailed questions. I don't know the first thing about diffuse large B-cell!'

He locked eyes with me for the first time, and nodded slowly with pursed lips. There was a long silence.

'Look, it's fine. I'll tell you everything you need to tell her.'

He sketched out a little mind map with all the drugs, when they would be administered, what their likely side-effects were, and then a larger box with some information about the cancer itself.

'And you can say that if she responds well to chemo, her chance of survival is around 80 per cent.'

'And if she doesn't?'

He looked up and off to the right.

'Best to not go there in this first consultation.'

'Right.'

'Okay, the third patient is Ms Nair. She has essential thrombocytosis. Her counts have been pretty stable on 500 of hydroxyurea. This is a six-month follow-up. The counts today all look good too, so just check she doesn't have any worsening symptoms suggestive of transformation to myelofibrosis, or that she doesn't have an enlarged spleen, then book her again in another six months.'

'And if she does have any of those things?'

'Just call me.'

'Professor, I don't mean to be rude, but wouldn't it be more efficient, and better for the patients, if you or one of your colleagues did the clinic, rather than giving a step-by-step guide to someone who has never done haematology before and is probably only here for a week?'

He sighed. 'Yes, probably. But I have to spend the morning booking next month's clinics. Our booker is away on maternity leave.'

'So *you* have to do that?'

He looked at me glumly. 'Someone has to, sport. We haven't found a replacement. You know, a decade ago I used to have a lot of free time to take the medical students for bedside teaching; often it would be the first time they had ever felt a spleen properly. I even used to organise teaching sessions for the registrars. It's hard to do that now — there's no time. The students don't get the same experience anymore. Half my day is spent on . . . codswallop!'

He gestured in the air with his right hand, then stared down forlornly at the ugly blue carpet.

'Anyway,' he continued, 'if I can figure out how to do a job that's not usually mine, so can you. Come on, clinic is starting in 10 minutes. Chop chop.'

My last patient of the haem clinic was in her seventies. She was accompanied by her daughter. She had a form of blood cancer and was on a second-line chemo treatment after first-line therapy had failed to get her into remission.

'So tell me, Doctor,' her daughter asked, 'why have you decided to go with [chemo option #1] as opposed to [chemo option #2]? I found some studies that say that [option 2] might be more effective.'

I opened my eyes wide and nodded at her slowly, desperately trying to figure out how to phrase my response to avoid looking like an idiot.

'Well, that is an excellent question. I can ask the supervising specialist, Professor Bond, at the end of this clinic. He'll be able to tell you more.'

She raised an eyebrow.

Too little too late, I thought.

'Okay, well, can you tell me why we can't get into the trial? Last time Dr Bond told us about this potential trial we could get into.'

'I'm not sure which specific trial you're referring to,' I said. Actually I didn't know about any trials, generally or specifically. 'But generally it's not possible to get into a trial when you're halfway through a course of chemo.'

'You don't really know much about any of this, do you?'

'No.' (Patients and families appreciate honesty.) 'I'll tell you what, why don't I get Professor Bond on the phone.'

For the rest of the consultation I stared at the floor with my phone on speaker on my outstretched palms while she talked to the professor.

◆◆◆

With the latest round of cuts to 'non-frontline' staff in 2024 the situation will get worse.

It's laughable for Health New Zealand to claim that the cuts will not affect frontline care.

11.

DEAR NURSE

It is nurses who actually take care of the patients. Any treatment I prescribe is quite useless without nurses to administer it to the patient, monitor them closely, attend to all their needs, prevent them from getting bedsores, stop them from falling over and breaking bones, and generally reassure them and keep them updated on what is going on.

Recently, I visited a ward to see a patient whose condition was getting worse, and who maybe needed to be admitted to the ICU.

I entered the central nurses' station, a boxed-in area with two small windows that peered out at the surrounding patient rooms. On one end of the station, neat rectangular cubbyholes were labelled by room number. They were where patient notes were supposed to be filed. In the classic contradiction of engineering functionality and human behaviour they were empty, and instead the station was strewn with patient notes and loose sheets of paper.

'Ms Daliwal. Ms Daliwal. Where are Ms Daliwal's notes?'

I wandered around like a lost duckling, glancing at the names written down the spines of the various folders. I barely took in the first few, as it is common knowledge that the folder you are looking for will always be the last one. Almost certainly it wouldn't even be in the nurses' station but on a trolley in a corridor somewhere, or in the medication room, or in the room of a different patient.

I was also looking for the patient's nurse, Kayla.

I was the only one in the nurses' station. I did a loop of the corridor around the station. No Daliwal file. No nurses. The whole ward appeared deserted. I started to wonder whether I had stepped through a portal and into a horror sci-fi where the Earth had become depopulated . . .

On my second loop, a nurse popped out of a patient's room. I jumped.

'Hey, you're not Kayla by any chance?'

'No. Haven't seen her for the last hour. Try rooms 18 through 26.'

'Okay, thanks. Where is everyone anyway?'

'Working.'

She strode away.

I poked my head into Room 18. An old man with wispy grey hair and sunken eyes looked back at me from his bed.

'Have you come to give me my pain meds?'

'Umm, no, sorry. Have you rung your bell for your nurse?'

He pointed above his head at the call bell light, which was on.

'Ah, right. I'm trying to find her too, so I'll send her your way as soon as I see her, okay?'

'Okay.'

Room 19 next.

'Who the fuck are you and what the fuck are you doing in my room, you rude little piece of shit!'

A Santa Claus lookalike with a red face and a large white beard appeared to be halfway through opening a cup of jelly when he saw me and unleashed this tirade.

I quickly ran out, since he looked like he was about to throw his jelly at me, and shouted over my shoulder.

'Sorry, just trying to find a nurse!'

I knocked on the wall beside the curtain in the next room.

'Is there a Kayla in there?'

'Yes, come in.'

Kayla was standing next to an old woman with a half-finished lunch tray.

'Sorry about our old mate next door,' she said. 'They can't control his aggressive behaviour at the nursing home and he's been throwing stuff at us all day.'

I nodded sympathetically.

'All right, Gillian, how about we try some of those medications now?'

She extended a pill cup towards the patient, who pushed it away like a two-year-old refusing her mashed carrot.

'I'm not taking your poison!' she said. 'It's all lies, all tricks!'

'Gilly, it's just your medications, to help you get better. How else will we get you home again if you don't take your pills?'

Gillian looked up at the nurse, narrowing her eyes and tightening her lips.

'And why would I trust you?'

I reflected that the story of Benjamin Button perhaps wasn't such a weird one.

Kayla sighed and looked at me. With reluctance, I launched into my pitch.

'My name's Ivor, I'm from the ICU. I've just seen Ms Daliwal—'

'Are you going to take her to the ICU?'

I saw a hopeful glint in her eyes.

'Well, I don't think there's much we can offer over and above what you're doing here, to be honest. Obviously she's got decompensated liver cirrhosis, but the main thing at the moment is her confusion. We can't do much about that and she doesn't really need any ICU supports. I feel she's best managed on the ward at this stage. Obviously if anything changes . . .'

I paused, as Kayla looked so deflated I feared she might suck the air out of me too.

'But it's very difficult for us to manage her,' she said. 'We're so short of nurses today, we're one to eight. I've got a patient next door who's been sitting in his own shit for the last hour because I haven't had time to change him . . .'

I recoiled at the image.

'. . . and these two keep going off, and Ms Daliwal keeps disconnecting her albumin infusion, and we're short HCAs [healthcare assistants] too. There's just no one to help.'

I picked at my teeth as I pondered her situation.

'Ms Daliwal is the sickest patient on the ward, and we can't really give her the treatment she's been prescribed because we just can't nurse her properly.'

'What's the nurse ratio on the ward supposed to be?'

'One to four.'

My eyebrows started upwards.

Kayla nodded at me.

God this stuff was difficult — stuff that seemingly didn't have anything to do with the practice of medicine. Ms Daliwal was not sick enough to need the ICU, which was filling up with patients as the day went on. If we brought in every patient like her, the ICU would be full faster than you could click your fingers. On the other hand, the patient clearly wouldn't — couldn't — get adequate care here. Then I considered that a doctor working in the Sudan probably had to deal with more difficult stuff than I did. Maybe, actually, all this had everything to do with the practice of medicine and I was too naïve to see it.

'Look, I know this really sucks. You're understaffed, and that's a problem we're not going to fix anytime soon. But we can't justify using up a scarce ICU bed because of that.'

'Fuck off with this poison!'

We turned back just in time to see Gilly hurl a pot of yoghurt in our direction. The creamy contents stretched out in mid-air in slow motion and landed on both of our scrubs with a comical splat.

Kayla turned back to me. White speckles hung off the strands of hair that fell down around her cheeks.

'You've got some on your beard.'

I stood with my hands still in my pockets.

'We'll take Ms Daliwal to the ICU.'

◆◆◆

Back in the intensive care unit I told the charge nurse to prepare for another admission.

'Another winner you've got here, Ivor.'

I shrugged.

I went to the tea-room, sat down and unrolled my ham and cheese sandwich. Next to me a frazzled-looking nurse was complaining bitterly to her friends about something. I eavesdropped.

'It's honestly crap — we're getting floated to the ED all the time these days!'

'I know. They're short of nurses down there every day. Last week they sent me down there and there was, like, one nurse covering all four resus bays.'

They shook their heads in unison.

'Well, today they decided to put me in triage. I've got all these patients coming in telling me, oh I've got abdominal pain, oh I hurt my leg, oh I've got a fever, and I'm like, "Okay, so what am I supposed to ask them next?" I'm not trained to do this. They don't even really explain the triage codes. It's honestly dangerous.'

'Yeah, and if something bad happens, you can bet they'll blame us, even though they made us do something we're not trained to.'

They all murmured in agreement.

Each type of nurse has a different set of skills. The emergency department and ward have been chronically short-staffed for years, and pulling nurses from elsewhere to fill in is becoming a regular occurrence now. There are few days when the emergency department is *not* short of nurses. This has created some perverse incentives: deciding to admit a patient to the ICU sometimes means we get to reclaim a nurse who has been pulled away.

I once took a shortcut through the triage bay, where ambulances deliver patients and a triage nurse allocates them an ED bed and an urgency ranking. The bay was gridlocked. One of my nurse friends was on triage. She looked flustered and sweaty.

'Are you okay?' I asked her.

'What does it look like?'

I winced. 'You look stressed.'

'I've got 12 patients here, and as soon as I find a bed for one, they bring another one in! It's just been me all day. This is fucking nuts!'

I pondered how to alleviate some stress.

'Want a bagel from the cafe?'

She side-eyed me and cocked her head down.

'I won't say no.'

Deteriorating working conditions are an addition to the crap nurses have to put up with.

A few years ago I was called to a cardiac arrest on the cardiology ward. A woman in her sixties had been on the ward after a large heart attack. She started experiencing worsening pain in her chest, then suddenly collapsed.

I turned up to find people spilling out of the door and shouldered my way through the crowd. Sometimes these things turn into spectator events.

Inside, a cardiologist was standing at the foot of the bed and leading the resuscitation. An anaesthetist who just happened to be walking by had inserted a breathing tube, and stood at the head of the bed pushing oxygen through it via an inflatable bag. Nurses were doing CPR and giving drugs. Another cardiologist beside the patient was tugging on a plastic tube that was sticking out between the patient's ribs.

'I'm from the ICU,' I said. 'How can I help?'

The second cardiologist looked up.

'The echo showed a large effusion [fluid or blood around the heart]; I've just stuck a drain in.'

The tube exiting from between the patient's ribs was draining fluid into a large plastic water jug that was wedged under the patient's armpit. Usually you would connect the drain to extension tubing, and then up into a proper closed container, but in the heat of the situation they had settled for the nearest available thing.

Bright red blood was filling the jug at an alarming pace.

'Right,' I said. 'Has anybody got a gas yet?'

'No.'

'All right, I'll try for that.'

I picked a syringe and a long needle off the IV trolley.

When a patient has no blood circulating around their body, the best place to get a blood sample is from one of the big veins passing under the fold between the torso and the thigh.

I placed my finger where I roughly knew the vein should pass and aimed the needle a centimetre below. The patient's whole body was shaking with every push from the CPR so it was hard to get a steady aim — the needle wobbled uncomfortably close to my finger. I cursed in my head. I did not want to accidentally stab myself with a dirty needle. Other than generating anxiety as you waited for the patient's HIV and hepatitis tests to come back, it created a mountain of paperwork.

I took a few deep breaths to steady my trembling hands, then stabbed quickly, pulling back on the plunger of the syringe. For a second it wanted to spring back to its starting position, but as I pushed the needle further in I felt the satisfying 'give way' of the plunger, and the syringe started to fill up with dark blood.

I turned to the IV trolley, protecting the needle with my other hand. I screwed off the needle and reached out with it towards the small yellow sharps container attached to the trolley.

I heard the yelp before I saw what happened. A nurse had reached across the IV trolley to hand something to another nurse, and our hands had crossed paths just at the wrong moment. A speck of blood hung off her index finger.

She pulled it close to her chest and held on to it with her other hand as we locked eyes. Hers were wide open and holding back tears. She gave me a silent look that implored me to take back what I had just done. I blinked a few times. All the noise around me was suddenly muted, and ice ran through my body to the bone. I opened my mouth to utter an apology but my mouth had dried up to the point I could not form words.

Tears started to well up in the nurse's eyes and she turned and fled the scene.

I handed off my blood sample and turned back to the patient.

Fuck, fuck, fuck.

There was nothing I could do to make this better right now. I had a patient in front of me and no choice but to push aside all the thoughts swirling in my brain.

The blood draining from around the patient's heart showed no signs of stopping. It had filled up four plastic jugs and it was still coming.

'I think she's ruptured,' said one of the cardiologists.

We all looked at the jugs of blood and nodded. A rupture is a devastating complication of a heart attack where the outer wall of the heart is so deprived of oxygen that it bursts. Unless you are in the operating room on a heart bypass machine, it is unsurvivable.

We called off the resuscitation efforts.

I sprinted out of the room and went to the charge nurse standing outside.

'Is everything okay?' she asked me, seeing the look on my face.

'Yes. Well, no. During the resus I accidentally gave one of your nurses a needlestick injury. I need to find her.

I don't know her name but she had black—'

'She's in the medication room.'

Inside I found the nurse sobbing, and a colleague had an arm around her shoulders. She looked up at me with swollen eyes.

'I am so, so sorry,' I said. 'I really didn't mean to do that. Are you okay?'

She smiled and nodded.

'It's okay. I know you didn't mean to.'

'I really should have been more careful. I've had a few needlesticks myself, so . . . well, I wish I had stuck myself rather than you.'

She smiled sadly.

I knew exactly what would be going on in her head. First you count the hours it will take to get the blood results back. Then you start to imagine the horror scenario where the patient comes back positive for HIV. The nauseating anti-viral medications you have to take in the hopes of avoiding getting infected. The six months of waiting to see if you will become HIV-positive. And if you do? They have good HIV drugs these days but sometimes the virus develops resistance to the drugs. Would you still be able to work? Would you still be able to have sex or find a partner? Who would you tell?

I jerked myself away from these thoughts.

'Have you had this happen before?' I asked her.

She shook her head.

'Okay, there's a standard procedure. I'll get someone to come and take your blood for testing — I don't think you want me stabbing you again,' I said, recoiling internally at the joke that was too soon. 'That's just to establish your baseline. The important thing is to test the patient, because if she's negative for everything, then there's nothing for you to worry about. There's a form you need to fill out to be sent with the bloods.'

'How soon do we get the results?'

'Should be by the end of the day.'

She nodded, looking more hopeful.

'All right,' I said, 'I'll go and get the samples from the patient.'

I jogged back to the patient's room. I froze at the entrance.

Shit.

Grief-stricken family were already standing around the bed, praying. I wasn't about to intrude on their grief by stabbing their loved one's dead body with more needles. But I wanted to get the samples away as quickly as I could. We couldn't use the blood I had taken during the arrest, because it needed to be sent in special blood tubes.

Suddenly I noticed the buckets of blood that had been tucked into a corner of the room. By some miracle nobody had yet disposed of them. A crazy idea came to me and I could feel myself start to breathe faster as I tried to think of any reason it wouldn't work. I came up with none.

I tapped a nearby orderly on the shoulder and said, 'Don't let anyone take those away! I'll be right back.'

I sprinted to the supply room and grabbed as many 50ml syringes as I could, then sprinted back. I dunked the first one in the bucket and yanked back on the plunger, worried that it might already have clotted off. There were some clots, but thankfully the tube filled up easily. I filled up the rest, and sent them to the lab. I called the lab to tell them what I'd done and make sure it would be okay. They confirmed that it would.

I breathed deeply and slowly once it was all done.

◆◆◆

On this occasion all the results were negative.

It's not as if nurses are getting stabbed by doctors left, right and centre. But they do the most patient-facing work and are the most exposed to all kinds of bodily fluids. They also cop the brunt of abuse from patients. I couldn't count the number of times I have seen nurses punched, kicked, scratched, or had their fingers crushed by patients grabbing them. Not to mention all manner of verbal abuse. Generally they don't report it because they say it won't change anything, or they don't have time to fill out more paperwork.

And who doesn't like a tweaked-out meth-head pulling down his pants and proclaiming, 'Bet you'd like some of this, bitch!' when you're at work?

Nurses also cop abuse from doctors. I'm ashamed to say I haven't been exempt from this behaviour. We like to think the world is divided into nice people and dickheads, but the reality is that everybody is balancing the level of stress they are facing with their ability to cope with that stress. Once the former exceeds the latter, a dickhead emerges. Every nice person has a dickhead inside; it's just the individual thresholds that vary.

Nowhere is the mismatch between stress and coping greater than when you first graduate from medical school. I recall my first night shift, and the feeling of being waterboarded with work. The pager alerts were coming thick and fast, and I felt as if I was trying to drink water from a fire hydrant. I had started at 10 p.m. and finally there was a lull at around 4 a.m., so I trudged up to the on-call room for my first break.

No sooner had I swiped to get in than I was paged to come and fill in a form to request a unit of blood for a transfusion I had just prescribed. The patient was on a ward on the other side of the hospital.

It was the drop that spilt the cup over. It was terrifying to experience how, in an instant, the part of my brain that stops you from doing things that are socially unacceptable went on holiday. I used the last of my energy to maintain a fuming pace all the way back to the ward. I filled out the stupid form, strode into the nurses' station and threw it at the nurse, saying, 'Next time tell me about this before I walk half the way to Timbuktu!'

By morning that part of my brain had returned from its travels and I returned to offer a sheepish apology.

Everyone in the hospital is stressed out and, as I've already observed, shit rolls downhill. The job is thankless, and the pay is better in Australia . . .

◆◆◆

Successive governments have reassured us that there is not a nursing workforce crisis. In 2024 we were told that the nursing workforce is increasing at a rate never seen before. The only data I can find in this regard comes from Nursing Council quarterly reports, which show that there were 9000 more new nurses with practising certificates in September 2024 than in September 2023, an increase of 12 per cent.

This sounds impressive, but hesitatingly I will point out that having a practising certificate does not mean you are employed, or even in the country. In fact, stories abound of nurses from overseas who obtain practising certificates only to arrive in New Zealand and find themselves jobless, even when jobs were previously promised to them. Health New Zealand's response to this is that many of the overseas nurses don't have the 'right mix' of qualifications for the jobs on offer here. So why were they promised jobs in the first place?

The same Nursing Council report shows that the proportion of certified nurses who trained in New Zealand (as opposed to overseas) is steadily falling. Meanwhile the proportion of internationally qualified nurses given New Zealand practising certificates who actually lived in New Zealand at the time their certificate was issued fell from 32 to 22 per cent in the year from September 2023. We don't know how many of the 78 per cent still living overseas had New Zealand jobs waiting.

But it's all okay. The Health New Zealand website tells us they have recently employed 3000 new FTE (full-time equivalent) nurses. On the other hand, their own workforce projections suggest that we are still 4500 FTE short. They go on to say that their own estimates of the shortage are 'clearly inaccurate' because the methodology is wrong, despite the same methodology being accepted for estimates in the doctor, paramedic, midwife, pharmacist and allied health professions.

Their justification? They have already decided that 'we have more generalist nurses than we need in New Zealand today, these greater number of nurses artificially amplify estimated shortages using our methodology'.

How could the people on the ground argue with this wonderful circular logic?

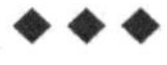

Some years ago I was on a night shift looking after a patient who had just had open heart surgery. Having someone stop then restart your heart is a big deal, and patients can get really sick before they get better. As a result, these patients often end up with tubes and lines sticking out of every orifice.

One of these is a catheter that runs through the jugular vein in your neck and sits inside your heart, where it measures the amount of blood your heart pumps around your body per minute. This is your cardiac output. In an average healthy human it is about 5 litres per minute but it varies a lot, depending on how much blood flow your body needs. When you exercise, your heart can pump more than 20 litres per minute.

Halfway through my shift I was walking around, checking up on patients. The ICU can be strangely peaceful at night, the gentle rhythmic hiss of a roomful of ventilators pushing air in and out soothing your nerves. The patients were all sedated and asleep, which meant there was no chance of a confused patient running around butt-naked (which was not uncommon in the ICU at night). One of my friends once told me that the first time he questioned his career choice was when he was about to inject a sedative into the butt cheek of a naked man who was pinned down by four security guards after spending half an hour being chased around the hospital.

Ms Jones was doing well after her surgery. Her numbers all seemed satisfactory, except her cardiac output was a little low, at 3.5 litres per minute. I frowned. This wasn't quite good enough, and the supervising specialist wouldn't be happy with me if I let it stay at that all night. I prescribed her half a litre of intravenous fluids. Hopefully this would fill up the heart more, allowing it to pump more blood around.

I came back half an hour later, expecting the problem to have gone away. Instead, the cardiac output now read 3.4 litres per minute.

I prescribed another half-litre of fluid. The patient's blood pressure went up, but still the cardiac output wouldn't budge. Now I was getting irritated. Why wasn't my therapy doing what it was supposed to do? Time for something more heavy-hitting. I prescribed a drug infusion to stimulate the heart muscle to squeeze harder. Within minutes the cardiac output had increased to 4.5 litres per minute. Quite pleased with myself, I went for a rest.

In the morning the specialist came around, and tore me a new one.

'What the fuck did you prescribe that for?'

'Well, the . . . the car . . . cardiac output was low,' I stammered.

'Are you a doctor or just someone who reads numbers?'

I didn't understand. I had just wanted to make the patient better. Why was I in trouble?

He looked at me and shook his head like a disappointed dad.

'It doesn't matter what the cardiac output is, only whether it is enough for the needs of the patient. Whatever cardiac output you have right now is enough for you, but it wouldn't be enough for someone running a marathon. Did Ms Jones, a sedated patient not doing any activity, have any signs that 3.5 was too low for her? Cold arms and legs, low urine output, was she unstable?'

'No.'

The lesson: absolute numbers are not the full picture. And so it is with numbers of nurses. It matters not how many we've employed; it only matters whether we have enough to meet the needs of the system. The answer, for anyone who has eyes and ears and has set foot in a hospital lately, is no.

In 2024 a multimillion-dollar extension was built in a major hospital, designed to increase elective surgery capacity, with thousands of extra surgeries promised. It opened six months late, and for even longer was bereft of patients — there were not enough nurses to staff it. Operating theatre staff as well as nurses were simply transplanted from the old building to the new. So much for extra capacity.

Nurses go on maternity leave, they retire, they resign, and the gaps they leave go unfilled. Local hospital managers no longer have the power to advertise or fill gaps. They have to go up the chain for approval. But of course we are 'over-budget', so nothing happens.

Numbers alone do not reflect experience. There is a huge difference between a pool of battle-hardened veterans and a pool of rookies. The loss of experienced and skilled nurses over the years has not gone unnoticed by the medical profession.

One contributing problem, aside from overwork, is the erosion of nursing independence.

On another of those fateful house officer night shifts early in my career, I had just lain down for a little rest when I got a message on the on-call phone app.

'Hi, Doctor, patient's chest drain suction has been prescribed in mmHg [millimetres of mercury], protocol says it needs to be prescribed in cmH2O [centimetres of water].'

I stared at the message through droopy eyelids, daring it to be a joke. After a few minutes, with no follow-up message of 'Haha, gotcha!', I fired back: 'You can google the conversion factor.' It was 1.36.

As soon as I shut my eyes, another beep wrenched them open.

'Okay, have googled. Is 600 cmH2O of suction correct?'

I tore out of bed so fast I practically teleported down to the ward. In the nurses' station a nurse was standing waiting for me.

'600 cmH2O of suction?' I said as I filled out the correct prescription on the chest drain protocol. 'Are you trying to suck his lungs out of his body? It's 25!'

He just smiled calmly at me.

'Okay doc, thanks for coming.'

He took the paper protocol and walked off.

I stared after him in incredulity, then started to laugh and shake my head as I realised I'd been played.

He knew full well how to convert between the two units. At the end of the day, though, if it wasn't prescribed on the protocol, it would be him that got in trouble for using his initiative, and the fastest way to get me down there was to seem incompetent.

This is the punitive and suffocating environment that nurses have to work in. The protocols and guidelines and forms that were designed to help, now enslave us all. People worry that not following a protocol to the letter means putting the patient at risk. There are always cases where the standard protocol is not appropriate, and you will not learn to recognise these situations and use your initiative if you always blindly follow the protocol.

Nurses' experience and judgement are being told to take a hike — the mighty protocol rules all.

When the Office of the Health and Disability Commissioner publishes its periodic case findings, nurses are always getting into trouble for this, regardless of whether or not their actions actually made a difference to the outcome of the case. Instead of encouraging independent thinking and problem-solving, our system punishes it. The result is enormous 'time rot', because now the nurse will page me when the patient complains of an itchy bum, because they are afraid to use their own judgement.

12.

PERSONAL RESPONSIBILITY OR SOCIETY'S PROBLEM?

A few years ago my dad mentioned to me that for the past few months he had been getting up several times at night to pee. Before he had finished talking I told him he needed to go see his GP and get his sugar checked. There's a test called the HbA1c, which gives an indication of your average blood-sugar levels over the preceding three months. Normal is less than 43. My father's was 100. He had a new diagnosis of diabetes.

'My GP said I need to lose some weight, and start taking a tablet of some sort,' he explained to me after his appointment.

I cocked my head sideways at him.

'This is really bad. Do you know your level was—'

'Yes, yes, more than twice normal, he told me.'

I narrowed my eyes.

'And did he tell you what would happen if you don't get this under control?'

'Remind me.'

'Diabetes damages your blood vessels. If you don't get it under control, eventually it will lead to heart attack or stroke. You'll go blind. You will start to lose nerve function in your feet and end up limping. Your kidneys will start to fail and you'll have to be hooked up to a dialysis machine. You'll die younger than you need to.'

He stared at me intently and tightened his jaw.

'Well, he did mention some of those things, probably not as brutally as you.'

'I'm your son; I can talk to you like this.'

'Is all that true or are you just trying to scare me?'

'I *am* trying to scare you, but actually it is all true. All those things could happen.'

He gulped. He nodded to himself while staring down at the ground.

'So how do I get on top of it?'

I pinched his belly.

'This. Get rid of this. Exercise every day. Stop snacking at night. Stop having so much sugar.'

He stared off into the distance, like a soldier having some kind of flashback.

'Okay. It starts tomorrow.'

I didn't expect what happened next. Overnight, the man cut his meal portions in half. He ate only at breakfast, lunch and dinner. He cut out all sweets, and he went for a long walk every day. He allowed himself a single slice of cake on special occasions, and I couldn't tempt him with a second even when I told him it would be okay just this once.

In six months he went from 105 kg to 79 kg. His HbA1c had come back to normal. Within a year he was off all diabetic medications, and still is several years later.

A lot of these chronic conditions are curable with the right lifestyle changes and if caught early enough. By definition, that makes them preventable too.

The problem is that I don't know many people who would be able to exert such incredible willpower. I certainly wouldn't. Being retired and getting a dog certainly helped.

Therein lies the problem with treating these conditions on a population level. Telling people to lose weight or change their lifestyle is generally not very effective. Changing habits is damned hard. So we cannot solely rely on GPs to turn things around.

◆◆◆

As a medical student on paediatrics I tagged along with some social workers doing home visits in South Auckland. One particularly wet day we were rolling through Ōtara in the fleet Mazda. I stared at the window, counting the drops of rain that zigzagged their way down the glass and hit the rubber join.

We were driving along a particularly narrow street. A man bundled up in a massive puffer jacket and socks and jandals was sitting under the cover of the superette, arms wrapped around himself and rocking back and forth. We passed the laundromat, then another dairy, then a clothing store. Further down the road, a monolithic red-and-white portrait of Colonel Sanders stood high above the intersection, seemingly surveying his subjects. It was the third KFC sign I had seen in the past half hour.

We turned off into a residential street that snaked its way into a cul-de-sac. A basketball hoop stood on one of the driveways, drooping down to the ground from where the base of the metal rim had cracked from rust.

All the houses looked the same. The top halves were clad in faded and cracked weatherboard, while the bottoms were concrete. Large wooden frames surrounded small square windows, weakened and warped over the years by the weather, and you knew the windows would only jerk open with a lot of effort. The roofs were nearly flat.

We were greeted by Mum at the front door. As soon as we went in, all I could think about was the warm heater inside the Mazda. The place smelt of clothes that had been left sitting wet in the washing for days. Black powdery streaks collected on the wall near the skirting.

We went and sat in the living room. I picked a spot on the sofa and leaned forward, arms close to my chest and one hand wrapped around my fist and tucked under my chin.

'How is Baby doing?' asked Maud.

Mum held the baby in her arms, feeding her a bottle.

'Yeah, good, good. Feeding better now. But we had to go into hospital last week. She got sick and she had to be in there for a day.'

'Oh no! What was she sick with?'

'A runny nose and breathing fast. She wouldn't eat anything.'

'Sounds like maybe bronchiolitis?'

Mum nodded and smiled uncertainly with the corner of her mouth.

'Well, anyway, good that she's better now. And how are the other kids?'

'They've all been sick too. I think Maisie might have got it from them.'

Two other kids sat playing in the corner of the room

next to a small heater. It was the only one I had seen. Green lights on the console indicated it was on, but even at the other end of the small living room you wouldn't know it.

The kids were aged four and five, but I only knew this because Maud had told me in the car ride over. Looking at them, you'd have put them a lot older because they were enormous. They looked the age of the 10-year-old brother who had just appeared and sat down to play with them.

'Before Baby was born, Mum and Dad were both working in the evenings, and Mr Ten was left to look after his brothers. Of course, he just went out and bought them McDonald's or other takeaways every night, because what else is a 10-year-old supposed to do?' Maud had explained to me.

'Isn't that illegal?'

'Well, yes, technically. What do you want to do — slap them with a fine?'

She eyed me up and down.

'Where did you grow up?' she asked.

'On the North Shore.'

'Hmm.'

This felt like a dig, and I looked over at her to confirm my suspicions but she just stared at the road ahead.

'A lot of what goes on out here may seem crazy to a lot of people, but it's just people making the best of a bad situation. Anyway, now Mum is obviously at home with the baby, and Dad is working two jobs, so he's hardly ever home.'

'How did you get on with asking the landlord about heat pumps?' Maud asked Mum. (This was obviously before the healthy homes regulations were introduced.)

'He said he'd get back to us, but it's been a month and we haven't heard from him.'

Maud frowned.

'Could we help you write to him? This place really needs to be sorted out. It's making you guys sick.'

Mum looked solemn.

'That would be great,' she replied.

She looked over at her oldest boy. He had rolled over on his back and the front of his shirt had lifted up. You could just make out the bottom of a scar that extended down the middle of his chest.

I was told that a couple of years earlier he had become sick with acute rheumatic fever. Rheumatic fever is an autoimmune disease usually contracted in childhood. It usually starts with a sore throat, although it can result from any infection with the bacteria Group A Strep (GAS) that goes untreated. It can cause serious, life-long damage to the heart. Mr Ten had been one of the unlucky children, most of them Māori and Pasifika, who needed open heart surgery to replace inflamed heart valves.

I thought back to the preceding weeks I had spent on the children's ward. I had been chatting to a junior doctor who had come over from England. She was telling me about life in the UK, and how she had come here to escape the falling debris in the rubble pile that was the National Health Service (NHS).

'It's been really interesting, the experience I've had in New Zealand,' she said. 'You get to see stuff like rheumatic fever, stuff English doctors only ever read about in a textbook.'

'What do you mean? You don't have any rheumatic fever?'

She giggled. 'Well, no, of course not.'

She looked perturbed that I didn't know this. I felt a flush fill my face. Here I was thinking we were so much better than the NHS, and yet we had this third-world illness on display for medical tourists to come and marvel at. I was seeing a new case of rheumatic fever every week!

Maud spent an hour at the house trying to figure out ways she could help. When we got back in the car I cranked the heater on full blast.

◆◆◆

Rheumatic fever happens almost exclusively in brown kids and New Zealand has a shameful record. It is a consequence of poverty and poor housing conditions. Cold, damp houses breed mould and are difficult to heat. People crowd together for warmth in houses that are already overcrowded, because they can't afford a bigger one. Mould and overcrowding lead to respiratory infection, asthma and strep throat. The cost and difficulty of getting to a GP mean these conditions often go untreated, and rheumatic fever is waiting in the wings.

Shitty rental houses are the root of the problem. A lot

have been poorly constructed, with no cavity behind the cladding, eaves that are too small, inadequate flashing on the windows, and no egress routes for water. This means the houses are not protected from moisture penetration, and a lack of insulation and concrete cladding makes them cold.

If you own your own home you have some incentive to fix these things to keep your family warm and dry. Making such improvements to your rental property, on the other hand, only cuts into your rental income. Fuck the poor, let them be happy with what they have, because of course they are the ones who occupy the poorest-quality rental housing.

The recent healthy home standards that were introduced in 2019 have gone some way to addressing these problems, but the deadline for landlords is July 2025 so we are in the dark as to what compliance has been like. Also, the regulations set out the bare minimum standards; we should be aiming higher.

Of course when it comes to poverty, one cannot have a conversation for long before two factions emerge. There are those who claim poverty is a choice; they say that those stuck in it need to work harder, make better decisions, and pull themselves up by their own bootstraps. They say that escaping poverty is a matter of personal responsibility. Their ideological opponents claim that everything falls on society's shoulders and it is only ever the system that is to blame.

◆◆◆

A 16-year-old named Angel came to us for heart surgery. She'd had rheumatic fever twice.

The heart has four valves — one for inflow and one for outflow, and one each for the left and right sides of the heart. Three of Angel's valves had been ravaged and she needed open heart surgery on all three. This was a massive undertaking in and of itself, but also her heart had started to fail; it wasn't able to pump enough blood around her body. Her kidneys had started to fail from lack of blood flow and she needed dialysis. Her obesity put extra strain on her heart.

It was going to be super-high risk to put such a fragile heart and body through the stress of stopping the heart for several hours and then restarting it, but it was her only option.

She came back from a long day in the operating room very unstable, although without all the tubes and lines sticking out of her everywhere she might have looked quite serene. She was sedated, her tummy gently rising and falling in time with the sigh of the ventilator. This is the state often described in the media as an induced coma. Doctors grimace at this technically inaccurate description.

The lines and tubes were all connected to a large monitor, whose squiggly red, green, yellow and blue lines flitted across the screen and told a different narrative. Numbers flashed and screamed for attention, and their shrill ringing would be silenced only to start up again a minute later. Doctors stood around the bedside staring anxiously at the monitor with hands in pockets, or stroking their chins. It was a great demonstration of the physician paradox: you really don't want your doctor to be taking this much interest in you.

The roller pumps of the dialysis circuit turned silently like the spindles of a cassette tape.

After several hours Angel stabilised. She was still the sickest patient in the intensive care unit, but things had settled down. Over the next several hours we performed the most difficult procedure in the ICU, one with its own five-letter acronym: MICLO. Masterful Inactivity and Cat-Like Observation. Sometimes you have to resist the temptation to fiddle too much and just let patients get better on their own.

Over the next few days her condition slowly improved. She went back to the operating room to have the bony part of her chest closed up fully; it is left open at the end of the operation when patients are really sick, to give the heart more room to work properly.

By this point Angel had swollen up like the Michelin Man. Her eyelids were tight and shiny and it was difficult for her to open them. The backs of her hands looked like softball gloves. Sodium-containing water had seeped out of her blood vessels and in under the skin from being so sick. We administered diuretics over the next few days trying to get her to reabsorb the fluid and pee it out.

Before anyone could count, seven days had gone by.

Angel woke up and could see us and hear us, but her muscles were so weak from seven days on a ventilator that all she could manage to move was her eyebrows. We replaced the breathing tube going through her mouth with a shorter tube that went straight into her neck, a tracheostomy, which would be more comfortable and allow her to be fully awake while waiting for her muscles to get strong enough so she could breathe on her own again.

Over the next several weeks she started to get her strength back. In the early stages after a tracheostomy patients can't talk, but Angel had a writing board. I learnt that her favourite artist was Dua Lipa. She loved reading fantasy books and she wanted to be a primary school teacher. She loved reading to her younger sisters and cousins, an excuse for them all to huddle together for warmth in the winter, growing up in a house in South Auckland like the one we had just visited.

Her family decorated the bedspace with photos of her home life. Looking at the group photos, I often couldn't recognise which one was Angel, and this is not uncommon with patients who have been seriously ill. Sometimes I don't want to know that this person once went to concerts, went to the beach, shared ham with family around the Christmas table, and smiled and laughed before all *this* happened.

It is an odd thing to come to know someone's personality through their eyebrows. She would dip the insides of them downwards, more deeply than I have ever seen anyone do, when you told her something she didn't want to hear.

'Sorry, Angel, we can't go outside today, it's bucketing down' or 'We can't let you have any food yet' or 'We need to do another session of dialysis today.'

She seized your gaze in this way and held it, stubbornly. I felt my stern doctor visage start to melt.

Behind it all she was just a scared teenager who desperately wanted to get better, and the things she wanted were what her idea of getting better looked like. Often, during long discussions among the medical team around the bedspace during rounds, I noticed her eyes darting between us, and her eyebrows taking on a pitiful quiver.

She would give me the 'sup' head nod every morning when I arrived and weakly wave at me with her arm close to the bed.

One day one of my terrible jokes happened to land and I saw the corners of her eyes crinkle up for the first time. She started coughing, which is the closest you can usually get to laughter with a tracheostomy in. She did the same when I told her she didn't need any more dialysis for now. It made my day immeasurably better.

One day when I arrived at work she wasn't doing so well. She had developed a chest infection and now she was sedated again, her eyebrows back to neutral. She was back on high doses of medication to support her blood pressure. Her heart was still very brittle, and wasn't coping well with the infection.

When playing basketball, and I imagine other sports too, you sometimes catch an opponent's elbow right in the middle of the chest. I'm sure most of you are familiar with the feeling of being winded, but in the heat of the game you don't let your opponent know they've hurt you. You walk it off, hoping nobody will notice, even as your lungs beg for a breath of air that never seems big enough.

So it is when these things happen. Even though it was a cloudless summer day outside, everything in the hospital seemed faded. I had piles of transfer summaries, admission notes and shift summaries to complete, like any other day, so I turned my attention to these. This is why you don't make friends with patients, I reminded myself. You end up casting a curse on them.

I spent all day jokingly referring to my friend, who was on shift with me, as Dr Death, because he always seemed to be around when bad things happened. I asked him if he was sneaking around injecting big doses of morphine into patients when nobody was looking. I told him that today we were employed by the ICU: the Ineffective Care Unit. I made him laugh. The more misanthropic and black I could make my jokes, the better I could hide my injury from my opponent — the faceless opponent that lurked the corridors in a black-hooded robe. Fuck you, I was telling him. You have no power over me.

To my deepening disillusionment, but not to my surprise, Angel got worse as the day went on. By the afternoon, her tummy had started to swell up. She was taken to the operating theatre, where the surgeons did what's known as a 'peek and shriek'. Inside her abdomen they found that most of the bowel was necrotic and dying from lack of blood flow. They closed her straight back up. She returned to the ICU where she died that evening, at the end of my shift, surrounded by family.

'How are you doing, man?' asked my friend as we walked towards the lifts.

'It's Friday,' I said, throwing my hands in the air and shrugging. 'Keen for a quick bevvy down the road?'

I rubbed my eyes in feigned tiredness.

You have no power over me.

◆◆◆

At times like this, all I see here is injustice, and all I feel is anger. I don't judge the decisions that Angel's family, and countless others like them, did or didn't make that landed them in poverty and kept them there. I'll leave that to morning talkback shows, where every caller is an expert; or to cognac-sipping armchair moralists who do little to address the injustice we see.

There are always people who lose out. Even if everybody put the same effort into life, there would always be a bell curve of outcomes. The only question is whether you think we should support the people who miss out or abandon them. The second point worth noting is that there is scarcely any event that has a single cause. You may know someone who made bad decisions that led them to where they are, and this may be a truth for that person, but that does not mean it is *the* truth in general.

What we see is a kind of outcome bias, where vices are viewed as character imperfections in the wealthy or clever, and as fatal flaws in those not so. You would be surprised to learn how many doctors who have been caught using drugs or alcohol on the job have managed to keep their jobs, and how sympathetic their colleagues are to their affliction. Would the petrol station worker down the road be afforded the same leniency? I am reminded of the famous passage from *King Lear*, which has stuck in my head ever since I first read it:

> *Through tattered clothes small vices do appear;*
> *Robes and furred gowns hide all. Plate sin with gold,*
> *and the strong lance of justice hurtless breaks;*
> *Arm it in rags, a pygmy's straw does pierce it.*

We know the cure. Higher disposable incomes, healthy housing and access to education. A key factor in this is parental income, which is the greatest predictor of poverty. The cure is the same no matter where you stand on the causes.

We have drifted a long way from the start of the chapter but it is all connected.

To reduce the burden on hospitals we must prioritise prevention and early treatment of disease. I talked earlier about the need for major changes in primary care.

But we also need to recognise that prevention is an

economic issue too. Poverty drives bad food choices. We need more regulation of fast-food advertising aimed at children, and the proliferation of fast-food joints in poorer suburbs.

Warm, dry housing is perhaps where we can do the most.

13.

LIFE EXPECTATIONS & THE BEST DEATH

Laughter helps us all. It is a soothing ointment on wounds that can never be healed.

I was called down to a trauma team activation. This alerts the on-call pagers for surgery, anaesthesia and intensive care so that everyone can convene on the ED resus bay, in preparation for an incoming trauma.

The ED doctor leads the team. The surgical doctor usually examines the patient for injuries, while ICU and anaesthesia help with breathing tubes, ventilators and organising an operating room.

We were told a gunshot injury was incoming. These are pretty rare in New Zealand, but more common in some places than others. A buzz filled the resus bay. We had no idea what we were in for. It might be as extreme as someone shot in the chest, in cardiac arrest, where we would need to open up the chest to expose the heart and carry out internal cardiac massage.

The buzz faded pretty quickly when our man arrived with the ambulance crew. He was sitting up smiling at us.

'Far, there's a lot of people here!' he said.

I was relieved, because I wasn't in the mood for too much drama that day.

We were told he'd taken a shotgun to the thigh, but didn't appear to have any serious bleeding and had stable vital signs. The team got to work. A nurse attacked him from the left and inserted an IV line into the crook of his elbow. Another came from the right and started hooking him up to all sorts of monitors. A third nurse was readying a bag of IV fluid. One by one his vitals flashed up on the ED monitor. The surgeon was busy examining his thigh. The ED doctor was conducting the well-rehearsed orchestra in front of her.

A plan was made for the patient to go to the operating room so the surgeon could explore the wounds. I stuck around for a bit to make sure he stayed stable and wouldn't need to come to the ICU. I came up close and peered down at his thigh. There was a single, round, fleshy hole in the front of it that went deep. The edge was scalloped. A bit of soot surrounded it and to one side the skin looked charred.

'Pretty trippy, huh?' said the patient, who seemed remarkably cheerful.

'Yeah. How did it happen?'

He looked down at his feet.

'Aww, you know. Just happened this afternoon.'

'Yeah, but who shot you?'

'Just happened at a party.'

'A party?'

'Yeah.'

'You got shot at a party?'

'You know how they get sometimes.'

I cocked my head at him while keeping eye contact.

'From the looks of this wound, whoever did it got up pretty close. Whose party was it?'

'My mate's.'

'Your mate's party? Who else was there?'

'Nobody. Just my other mates.'

'So one of your mates shot you?'

He paused for a second and tightened his lips.

'Yeah,' he said.

'I think you need better mates.'

We stared at each other for a second, then both burst out laughing.

I knew he was full of shit. He knew I knew he was full of shit.

I suppose you have to have a certain sense of humour to survive the gang lifestyle. You have to have a certain sense of humour to see people shooting, stabbing and running each other over and not despair at the hopelessness of it all.

I thought of all the patients who complain about the hospital coffee, or the uncomfortable beds, or the wait times, and how they couldn't be more different to our shotgun victim. You could probably mess up his care pretty badly and he still wouldn't complain. It's all about expectations. If you are used to getting everything you want, nothing is ever up to standard. If you are used to existing on the bare minimum, even simple things can be a luxury.

Expectations are central to a good career in medicine. If you go to medical school hoping to save lives, become well-respected and get rich, you will sober up quite quickly. If you're after a job that sucks your time, youth and patience but is mostly rewarding and has some job security, then you will be okay.

My own pathway into medicine was somewhat accidental. Having said to myself throughout high school that I would never go to medical school because I didn't want to take tests for the rest of my life, I found myself at the end of seventh form (Year 13) with no clue what I wanted to do. My parents suggested that, being good at science and not too bad with people, I should reconsider medicine. I thought that sounded reasonable.

I was a bumbling medical student. On one rotation with the neonatal team I attended a high-risk birth with the specialist nurse practitioner. The baby emerged looking okay, and we began the quick newborn exam and vitamin K shot. (All newborns are given this as they are deficient in vitamin K, which can lead to bleeding in the brain.) The nurse practitioner asked me to draw up the vitamin K while she examined the baby. I took up the needle and syringe and the tiny vial of K.

'You want to give the shot?' she asked once she was done, not looking at me. When there was no reply she looked up and darted her head side to side.

'Where did our medical student disappear to?'

The midwife shrugged her shoulders.

I emerged from the patients' bathroom holding my finger wrapped in layers of paper towels, stained bright red.

The nurse practitioner leaned towards me, motioning with her open palms.

I gave my meek confession.

'I stabbed myself.'

'I can see that. Where is the vitamin K?'

'Most of it is in my finger.'

'Okay, we'll get another one.' She was desperately trying to suppress a smile.

My skills didn't improve. Not long after that I spent a day shadowing a doctor at the sexual health clinic. While we were waiting for a patient to arrive she pulled out a plastic penis from a cupboard and stood it on the table, shaft pointing towards the ceiling.

'Simple education goes a long way,' she said, handing me a condom packet. 'Condoms are really effective prevention. Why don't you demonstrate how to do it?'

I stared at her. Was she was joking, or just really passionate about teaching effective contraception? Was I perhaps entering some adult film situation that I did not want to be a part of? Her lined face was inscrutable.

I timidly took the packet from her and went to tear it open, but my hands were sweaty and I couldn't grip it properly. I tried the other side. The doctor coolly watched me struggle for a minute before remarking in a flat voice, 'Boy, imagine how much harder it would be in the dark.'

I know I went red as ketchup.

I didn't seem to thrive under pressure. It was therefore a total surprise to me that I drifted towards intensive care. Where you end up is often a function of which personalities you gel with, and every specialty has its own personality type. I'm not sure what it says about me that ICU doctors have a reputation for being arseholes and annoyingly anal-retentive.

I had thought that getting into medical school would be the big barrier and everything after that would be sweet. Then I encountered the stress of trying to get the jobs I wanted and get into specialty training. Once I had the first set of specialty exams behind me I could relax, I told myself. Then there was the next set of exams.

I realised the rest of my life would consist of waiting to jump the next hurdle — waiting for the right job to come up, for retirement, for death — if I didn't learn to stop and smell the roses along the way.

What this job has taught me is that life is fickle. At any moment you could be struck down by an aneurysm bursting in your brain, by a falling tree, or by the flu. You would think this would make you slow down and savour every moment. You would think that this would help you recognise the things that truly matter. Nobody in their final moments tells you they wish they had mended fewer relationships. Nobody says they wish they spent more time working and less time with the people they love. Nobody says they wish they were richer.

But you continue to sweat the small stuff. You swear at people who cut you off in traffic. You continue to start arguments about how to load the dishwasher. You insist on holding grudges. You worry about whether it's going to rain tomorrow or whether your flight is going to be delayed. You worry about what other people think of you. This is the human curse that we have to endure. When our brain sees a reality that is too difficult to confront, it simply throws an invisible cloak over it. In this case it is the smallness, the unimportance, the fleeting nature of our lives.

◆◆◆

At the end of a typical day I am called to assist with a resuscitation on the ward. I arrive to find the emergency response team in the thick of delivering CPR.

I look past the medical notes that someone shoves in my face, past the team leader bellowing instructions like a drill sergeant, past the syringes of drugs being drawn up and lying around, and I look at the patient.

He is very old and frail. I see the gaps between his ribs. I see wisps of white hair sticking up from his head. With every two-handed push on the middle of his chest, at 100 times a minute, I hear a crunching sound, and his ribs are caving in like a collapsing tower of cards.

'What is his resuscitation status?' I ask the team leader.

'Not documented.'

I breathe deeply. Of course. When you are under-resourced there is simply no time to spend having in-depth conversations with patients about what they envisage at the end of their lives. Does this patient actually want us performing these heroics? Would he rather be allowed to slip quietly away?

One of the doctors suctions inside the patient's mouth, and bright red blood fills up the inside of the plastic catheter. There is blood on the floor from where a new IV line has been inserted in his arm. The room is a mess of plastic wrappers, discarded equipment, bodies bumping into and shouting at each other and the cables of the defibrillator running haphazardly through the middle of it all.

You can tell quite quickly whether CPR stands a chance of working. The person still looks kind of alive. I recalled all the times in my career that I had certified a death. You go through a detailed process to make sure: checking the pupils, checking the pulse, checking for breathing. But you pretty much know within one second of looking at them. They just look dead. You just know, without knowing how you know, that their 'spirit' has left their body. People who look like this during CPR don't make it back.

We eventually stop resuscitation efforts. The patient's wife has been in the room watching the entire time. This is the memory she will have of her dearly beloved's last moments.

CPR when done properly is violent. You have to push hard because you are pushing on the heart through the chest wall. If you don't break some ribs, you're probably not pushing hard enough.

It doesn't take very long without good blood flow for the brain to start undergoing irreversible damage, and all the other organs in the body also suffer. The body has to run a marathon, and getting the heart restarted is only the first 21 km. It then has to recover from the shock and stress of what has happened, and try to breathe effectively with broken ribs.

Not everyone is capable of running a marathon. Shows

like *ER* and *Grey's Anatomy*, and a million and one carbon-copy TV dramas, depict events that bear little resemblance to reality. A terribly good-looking (but personally flawed) doctor steps up and saves the day with amazing CPR, and then spends the rest of their shift with their hands in their pockets wistfully staring through the window of the recovering patient's room (because of course they have no other work to do). The patient makes a miraculous recovery and returns to normal life a few days later.

Back on planet Earth, the survival rate of CPR is only one in ten. This is for the average person. For someone old, frail or unhealthy it is much lower. And this is survival we are talking about. You may 'survive' but end up as a vegetable.

Doctors perform CPR when there is more chance of doing good than harm. To do good, the patient has to be strong enough to cross the finish line of the metaphorical marathon. But it also depends on why their heart has stopped. If the heart is the first organ to stop — for example they are at the shopping mall and a heart attack disrupts the electricity within the heart — then there is a chance of restarting it and fixing the problem that made it stop in the first place. If the heart stops after other organs are already compromised — for example the patient is sick in hospital with flu and their condition is deteriorating — then it is like trying to restart an engine that's out of petrol.

How can you possibly harm someone who is already dead, you might ask? Isn't CPR always worth a try? Think of it another way. When death seems certain, we have the power to control how it happens. People's last memories of their loved ones can be of a peaceful and dignified death, surrounded by family, soft music and perhaps prayer. Or they can be of medical staff unceremoniously abusing their loved one's corpse, breaking bones and spattering blood on the floor.

Death is a natural part of life, so why make it unnatural? CPR can also actually harm the patient. Sometimes the procedure succeeds in getting enough blood flowing to the brain that the patient recovers a bit of awareness. I have seen people move their arms during CPR, and I have seen patients who have survived (who belonged to the group who were good CPR candidates) who could recall what staff were saying during the resuscitation. Is this what you would want for your last experience of life on planet Earth?

There was an outcry in the UK during Covid when it was discovered that doctors were making do-not-resuscitate (DNR) decisions for patients. Every so often the news media in New Zealand run articles about heartless doctors who refused to resuscitate someone's family member. But this is the way the law works. (Having a DNR only means CPR won't be performed; it does not say anything about other treatments.)

In New Zealand, the final decision about whether a treatment is indicated is up to the medical professionals. I'm not going to offer chemotherapy to someone with the flu, because it's not going to do any good. I'm not going to offer CPR to someone where it's not going to do any good. 'Good' means there's a reasonable chance of getting through and ending up in a state that they would find acceptable. It's good practice to ask patients (if possible) and families what they would like, but at the end of the day it is not their decision. This is not doctors 'withholding life-saving treatment' or 'playing God'.

On the rare occasion that a doctor has time to discuss the issue properly with a patient, many will say that CPR is something they absolutely would not want. But where in the Sisyphean day of a hospital doctor lugging the crumbling system around on their backs can they find the space to sit down and explain such things properly? Even if the decision is clear, we like to talk to people before we document a DNR. When the emergency team arrives to an unfamiliar patient without a resuscitation status documented, they will initiate CPR until further information is obtained. It might soon become clear that CPR is not appropriate, but by then it is too late. There are a lot of people getting CPR who probably wouldn't have wanted it. The overwrought system is depriving people of the chance of a dignified death.

We are uncomfortable with talking about death, yet it is as natural, as unavoidable and as significant as our birth. The medical profession is often just as bad. I was taught to always explicitly use the words 'death' and 'dying' when having difficult conversations with people; you want to be crystal clear in your meaning. You don't want to hide behind euphemisms about passing away, or slipping away. Yet, still, every time I go to say the word I feel my voice faltering. There's a split-second break in my cadence that is imperceptible to anyone else. Our conditioning runs deep.

◆◆◆

When I was in my final year of medical school my grandpa started to get more unsteady on his feet. He had always struggled, because of nerve damage from his diabetes, but now he had fallen three times over the course of a week. My grandma mentioned that she had noticed his tummy was swollen and firm. I knew immediately what was probably going on but I didn't say anything, and I didn't offer to examine him. I secretly hoped Grandma wouldn't take him to hospital because I knew no good could come from it, but after the third fall when he couldn't get up she called an ambulance.

A scan showed his abdomen was full of cancer. There was so much of it, it was impossible to tell where it had originated from. I wondered how we had all missed the fact that he was so sick. These things don't develop overnight. I was disappointed in myself. What was the point of my six years of medical education?

What I have seen since is that people get by and get by until they don't. It's amazing how damaged and destroyed the chassis can get, yet it keeps on rolling through the streets in neutral until the wheels fall off.

Grandpa was always irreverent when it came to his

health. He was a diabetic who had a second and third helping of cake at family gatherings, and he passed on the sweet-tooth gene to me. His doctor had told him many years ago that he needed to cut back or it would kill him.

'I eat sugar, and it eats me. Seems fair,' he replied.

As much as I wanted to tell him off, I couldn't help but respect this.

He loved to pull your leg. If you were a spider, he'd pull all eight of them. He would always remind me that it was a huge mistake to get married before you were 25, but you shouldn't wait much past 30. He told me stories of being a nurse in the countryside in Yugoslavia and accepting plum brandy as payment, and having to sharpen needles in the evening for re-use.

In hospital he seemed to age about five years in the course of a few days. There is something about the faded hospital gowns — the way they are always somehow too loose around the neck but too tight around the shoulders where the buttons come together; too tight around the belly but always leaving the nether regions at risk of flapping in the breeze. The fluorescent lighting contributes to the sallow and infirm look. The scruffy beginnings of a beard added to this. I started to worry for the first time that he wouldn't make it to my graduation in a few weeks' time. He'd been talking about it the whole year.

One day I arrived and his bed was missing. His doctors had sent him down for a biopsy of the mass in his abdomen, to figure out what type of cancer it was. I had steam coming out of my ears. Fuck my profession and their one-track minds. What was the point? We all knew he didn't have long left — there was no treatment possible. I wanted him to be able to come home to die with hospice care, which would take a bit of organising. Instead he was in a dungeon somewhere in the radiology department, being tortured by a doctor with a long needle. They spent a few hours trying and in the end couldn't get any samples.

The next night he died peacefully in his sleep in his hospital bed.

I spent the next few weeks imagining an alternative reality where we had never taken him to hospital. Knowing how sick he was, we took him either to my parents' house or my auntie's place. We took turns looking after him until the same thing happened, but without ill-fitting hospital gowns, long pointy needles and fluorescent lights. Only shafts of sunlight streaming in between rows of blinds, the wind stroking the fur of the lamb's-ear leaves out in the garden, and the tūī in the trees singing their song.

The hospital is still a common place for people to die, but it doesn't need to be.

Many years later we had a patient called Ariki, who was dying in the ICU. As horrible as a hospital is to die in, the ICU is 10 times worse. In this case the relationship between the family and the doctors had not been perfect, but for some reason they liked me.

We had removed his breathing tube. The patient's sister beckoned me to the room, where Ariki was awake but sleepy. A tiny high window let in a sliver of light, though not enough to dispel the gloom that hung in the room.

'We want to go home,' she said.

I misunderstood. 'Well of course, you guys can come and go as you like. Only I don't know how much time you have.' I tried to nod subtly towards Ariki.

The sister laughed at me.

'No, you don't understand. He wants to go home. We want him to come home. Home to die. Not here.'

'Oh. Right. Well, I don't know how we would do that. It takes a lot of organising for things like this. I don't think we've ever done it straight out of the ICU. We'd need to organise his medications—'

'We can give those if you show us how.'

'Okay. Let me go and ask some people.'

'I'm sure you'll be able to figure out a way.' She smiled politely at me and went to sit down next to Ariki and hold his hand, leaving no doubt that the conversation was over.

My boss, Kenneth, and I agreed that this probably wasn't a good idea.

'You want to go and tell her?' I asked.

'No,' said Kenneth, 'she doesn't like me very much. Why don't we just . . . I dunno . . . why don't we just try? We'll just call an ambulance and his nurse can go with him.'

'I'm pretty sure they won't want to go without a doctor.'

'Why don't you go?'

'I'm holding the emergency pager!'

'Well, Emily can hold it for a few hours.'

'Is this the best use of my time?'

'Probably not.'

'I'm not even sure he'll make it that far. What if he dies on the way? I can't just drop off a dead body at the house.'

'Why not?'

'I dunno. It just doesn't seem right. I'd have to call the GP and ask them to come and write the death certificate, even though he died under our care.'

'Yeah, I suppose that doesn't look so good.'

We sat in silence for a moment.

'I'll tell you what,' Kenneth said. 'How about we make it clear to the family that if he dies on the way, you'll have to turn around and come back. Just make sure he keeps his oxygen on until you get there, then they can take it off. Be clear that there is a good chance that might happen, and they need to be okay with it. Dying in the ambulance might not be exactly what they had in mind.'

'I think at this point they are thinking anything would be better than here.'

I sat in the back of the ambulance as we rocketed down chip-seal streets lined with potholes, weaving through traffic. We were going lights and sirens by my instructions. I didn't know if there were protocols dictating which situations were appropriate for such speed, and if there were I found it hard to believe that this was covered. But the ambo hadn't protested, so I tried not to think about it.

I had a slight worry that all the jostling would be a bit too much for Ariki's body to handle. The wind whipped my hair through the small sliding window I had opened just above me, and, despite fearing that we would tip over at every corner, it was hard to not feel kind of relaxed being part of the raw outside world while my colleagues were trapped in the sterile maze of the hospital. I had no phone or pager to worry about, and one patient in my care whom I couldn't make any worse.

We pulled up to the house where the rest of the family were waiting for us. I went to open the back door of the ambulance but the family waved me away. I got out through the front instead.

'Is everything okay?' I asked them.

'He wants to go to the beach.'

'The beach.'

'He's been a sailor all his life, and he wants to die next to the ocean.'

'That wasn't part of the arrangement.'

His sister looked at me so sharply I felt I had a gun to my head.

'What's it going to cost you?' she said. 'Come on, it's only 10 minutes down the road.'

I looked over at the ambulance officer, who shrugged his shoulders.

'Okay, okay. But what is he going to sit or lie on? We have to take the stretcher back.'

'Don't worry, we'll sort it out.'

We pulled up to a little beach tucked away at the end of

a side street. A playground stood off to one side, children swinging on the monkey bars, and a grassy area led to the sand, with a narrow pathway cutting through it. Cliffs bounded the small beach area, with houses at their tops, and pōhutukawa grew from the rock face and hung down over the shore, their red spindly flowers in full bloom.

We trundled along the uneven pathway while the kids in the playground stared. A couple of burly family members carried a large sofa between them. We got down to the sand and lifted Ariki out of the stretcher and onto the sofa, placed under the shade of a pōhutukawa and facing the sea.

'How will you get home?' I asked his sister.

'It's okay. We have a van, and some muscle.' She looked over at the guys who had carried the sofa, who nodded their heads upwards and smiled. She looked back at me and smiled kindly. 'But I don't think he has that long.'

I went back to the hospital.

Ariki died at the beach later that afternoon, sent off with a gentle guitar and a chorus of family.

I often remember that day and think that it is the most meaningful care I have ever been able to provide.

I have not been able to replicate this for any patients since. All the stars aligned on that day, and we all went out of our way to do something we were not set up to do.

I see too many patients die in hospital while waiting to go to hospice or home. Hospices, like every other damned health-related thing, are underfunded. They receive less than half of their funding from the government and are struggling to stay viable. They rely heavily on donations, community fundraising, and income from their op shops. Of course when the economy is in crisis, these sources dry up.

The costs of hospice care are rising exponentially, and faster than inflation, which is unsurprising when you consider the growth in our old and chronically sick population. Perhaps this is why in 2024 New Zealand was in twelfth place in the *Economist*'s Quality of Death Index, having been third in 2015.

14.

SOME HARD DECISIONS NEED TO BE MADE

If you've made it this far, I thank you for reading. While a lot of my anecdotes were written to entertain, they all of course contribute to a deeper message.

The message is that New Zealand's hospital system is in crisis.

- We need more registrars, more specialists, more nurses, more wards, more operating theatres and clinics and better IT. We need to be investing rather than limiting funding and cutting roles.
- The ageing and increasingly unwell population is rapidly growing, faster than our ability to look after it.
- The shortage of doctors will not be addressed in any satisfactory way by just increasing medical student numbers or blaming the Australians. We need to address the bottleneck of registrars wanting to transition to specialists, utilise our specialists more efficiently, become more competitive with other countries, and create a better-resourced environment that doesn't burn out local or foreign doctors.
- We need to better fund hospice care and social/ care services in the community that will help save hospitals for what they do best: looking after really sick people.
- Poverty and substandard housing quality need to be addressed as priorities.
- Doctors need to lose the mobster mentality that

keeps bullies and sociopaths in positions of power within the medical profession.

- We need to find a way to regulate the perverse incentives that concentrate high-quality care in the private sector at the expense of the public sector.
- Doctors need to communicate more honestly with the public.

None of these problems will be fixed while politicians and administrators bury their heads in the sand and deny that there is a healthcare crisis. Government-mandated targets do not make up for a lack of healthcare investment. Cutting 'behind the scenes' services is shooting yourself in the foot.

Patients also need to realise that medicine is an art as well as a science, and that while doctors and nurses will do their utmost, they are not super-human.

There is money in the government coffers: New Zealand is a first-world country. It is a question of priorities. Investing in the future health of our population at large would come back to society tenfold. If we are not investing, we are destroying.

With the right therapy and lifestyle changes, the condition is still reversible. It is up to all of us.

ACKNOWLEDGEMENTS

My thanks to the following people for their help with this book.

Michelle, Leanne and the rest of the team at Allen & Unwin for allowing me to tell my story. Freelancers Rachel, Mike and Teresa for editing and proofreading. Megan for the book design, and Stephen for taking the cover photo.

Emma and Dave for providing advice and contacts to an aspiring writer.

David and Nicola, my high school English teachers, who taught me to show, not tell.

My friends and colleagues who agreed for their stories to be included in the book.

Patients and their families who gave consent for their experiences to be shared, as well as those whose stories

I have anonymised. You have all taught me so much over the years.

My family — those still here and those departed — who have always supported me and been an inspiration.

Lastly, my beautiful wife, Sarah, who is glad I can focus my attention back on her now!

ABOUT THE AUTHOR

Ivor Popovich works in Auckland as an intensive care doctor and will fully qualify as a specialist in August 2025. He has worked across different hospitals and specialties since finishing medical school in 2015. When not at the hospital he can be found shooting hoops or tickling the ivories on his piano.